PRAISE FOR
THE SLEEP-DEPRIVED TEEN

"In this timely book, Lisa L. Lewis underscores why sleep is so vital for adolescent well-being and resilience and offers detailed, actionable tools for bringing about change. Grounded in science and filled with insights and inspiration, *The Sleep-Deprived Teen* is a call to action for parents everywhere to help their teens thrive."

—**Arianna Huffington**, founder & CEO of Thrive Global

"In her compelling and deeply researched book, Lisa L. Lewis shows why sleep matters to the physical, emotional, and social well-being of teenagers. She deftly reviews the science, then provides practical advice for putting those scientific insights into action. For parents and educators everywhere, this book is an urgent and timely read."

—**Daniel H. Pink**, #1 *New York Times* bestselling author of *When*, *Drive*, and *The Power of Regret*

"Lisa L. Lewis' book should serve as a wake-up call to parents, lawmakers, school administrators, coaches, and teens everywhere. It's nearly impossible to convince adolescents they need more sleep, but this book is full of persuasive facts even the most exhausted teen might heed. Don't let your aspiring NBA players miss the chapter on sleep as a competitive advantage! *The Sleep-Deprived Teen* is a bright and easy read with profound implications for the health and development of teens."

—**Michelle Icard**, author of *Fourteen Talks by Age Fourteen*

"*The Sleep-Deprived Teen* is a must-read for anyone caring for tweens and teens. It explains in a clear and accessible way how kids' sleep patterns change during puberty and why good-quality sleep is so critical to the physical and emotional well-being of our adolescents."

—**Vanessa Kroll Bennett**, cohost, *The Puberty Podcast*

"*The Sleep-Deprived Teen* provides a conversationally paced review of the scientific background behind teen sleep challenges and outlines a roadmap for healthier and better-slept teens through community and school advocacy. Investing in today's teens, who are tomorrow's leaders, truly does start with a good night's sleep!"

—**Maida Lynn Chen, MD**, director of the Sleep Center at Seattle Children's Hospital and professor of pediatrics at the University of Washington School of Medicine

"Filled with outstanding research and reporting, *The Sleep-Deprived Teen* should convince every parent and educator of teens to make healthy sleep a priority. Lisa L. Lewis covers the latest research on sleep-deprivation and compels readers to consider practical changes around school start times, sports practices, media use, caffeine, driving habits and more, all with a goal of improving teen health and engagement with learning. Read it with your teen today!"

—**Denise Pope, PhD**, cofounder of Challenge Success and senior lecturer at Stanford University Graduate School of Education

"While we often view waking sleepy teens for pre-dawn school as a joke at best or an annoyance at worst, *The Sleep-Deprived Teen* shows why this practice undermines the health and well-being of children, families, and entire communities. Whether you live with, work with, or even know any teenagers, this engaging, illuminating book will awaken you to this 'sleeper' of an issue and show you how we as a society can address it."

—**Terra Ziporyn Snider, PhD**, executive director and cofounder, Start School Later

THE SLEEP-DEPRIVED TEEN

THE SLEEP-DEPRIVED TEEN

WHY OUR TEENAGERS ARE SO TIRED, AND HOW PARENTS AND SCHOOLS CAN HELP THEM THRIVE

BY LISA L. LEWIS, MS

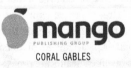
mango
PUBLISHING GROUP

CORAL GABLES

For permission requests, please contact the publisher at:
Mango Publishing Group
2850 S Douglas Road, 4th Floor
Coral Gables, FL 33134 USA
info@mango.bz

For special orders, quantity sales, course adoptions and corporate sales, please email the publisher at sales@mango.bz. For trade and wholesale sales, please contact Ingram Publisher Services at customer.service@ingramcontent.com or +1.800.509.4887.

The Sleep-Deprived Teen: Why Our Teenagers Are So Tired, and How Parents and Schools Can Help Them Thrive

Library of Congress Cataloging-in-Publication number: 2022932267
ISBN: (print) 978-1-64250-791-1, (ebook) 978-1-64250-792-8
BISAC category code HEA046000 HEALTH & FITNESS / Children's Health

Printed in the United States of America

For sleepy teens everywhere

CONTENTS

FOREWORD

There are times when one person can spark a tremendous change. One such spark is the story of how Lisa L. Lewis helped improve the sleep health of millions of kids.

For over twenty years, I was aware of the increasing data that our adolescents were systematically being sleep-deprived by society, and that the school system was one of the biggest drivers of this problem. I could recite the literature that stated that delaying school start times would improve the health of our children. I spoke about it many times over my career. But even after having spoken at several schools, I too had grown cynical that we could make a change. Although the audience was always interested in the information, they inevitably would politely say they were powerless to make any changes or that the science did not apply to their communities.

You can imagine how surprised I was to learn that a bill had been introduced in my adopted home state of California by State Senator Anthony Portantino to delay school start times to help adolescents get more sleep. I was even more surprised when I learned that he introduced the bill after reading a commentary Lisa had written, "Why School Should Start Later in the Day," which ran in the *Los Angeles Times* in September 2016. One of the many facts that resonated with him was how sleep deprivation can be a factor in suicidal behavior, given that a close family member of his had died by suicide.

That state bill, which called for the public high schools and junior high schools in California to implement healthier starting times, was quickly defeated in Sacramento. But the spark was lit. Senator Portantino vowed to work through the legislative process to reintroduce the bill. The second time around, the bill made it out of the legislature only to be vetoed by the governor. Undeterred, and with a growing coalition of supporters and increasing scientific data, he introduced the bill for a third time.

We worked together throughout the journey as part of a collective effort by a small, dedicated group of volunteers, including Joy Wake and others in Sacramento who regularly called on legislators to share the peer-reviewed research and other updates. In 2019, our efforts culminated in California being the first state in the nation to pass a law of this scope protecting adolescent sleep health.

No fundraising was ever done in support of this bill, and it was up against some of the most powerful lobbyists in the state. Indeed, many political experts expected the bill to be defeated. But science won out.

In my practice I've seen countless teens over the years whose sleep issues are hindering their health and well-being. With this book, parents now have a clear, accessible guide about the importance of sleep health for their adolescents and the far-reaching ramifications it can have.

–Rafael Pelayo, MD, FAASM, clinical professor, Sleep Medicine
Division, Stanford University School of Medicine

INTRODUCTION

Is your teenager well rested?

If you're reading this, chances are the answer is no.

That's stressful for both of you. And, as a parent of teens, I know it's not easily solved by saying, "Go to bed!"

I'd like to point out that you're not alone: Unfortunately, this sleep-deprived scenario has become the norm.

★ ✦ ✦

In 2007, when the Centers for Disease Control and Prevention (CDC) first added teen sleep to its national Youth Risk Behavior Survey, only 31 percent of high schoolers said they got at least eight hours of sleep on school nights.[1] By 2019, that was down to 22 percent.[2]

In fact, eight hours is the *minimum* amount they need: The National Sleep Foundation recommends that fourteen- to seventeen-year-olds get eight to ten hours a night. (This drops to the adult range of seven to nine hours at age eighteen.)[3]

Teens themselves know their sleep falls far short of this. As Jessica Lahey recounts in *The Addiction Inoculation*, her 2020 book about preventing teenage substance abuse, "When I tell adolescents how much sleep they are supposed to get, they laugh. Whole auditoriums full of middle and high school kids just throw their heads back and laugh. Their message is clear: teens get nowhere near enough sleep."[4]

Not only does teen sleep loss have important implications for substance use, as Lahey discusses in her book, it's worrisome for a number of other reasons.

Sleep-deprived teens are more likely to engage in risky behaviors and be anxious, depressed, or suicidal. At school, their grades are affected, and they're absent or tardy more often. Sleepy athletes have a greater risk of injury, and drowsy teen drivers are more likely to crash.

The changed sleep rhythms of adolescence are a driving factor. But there are also societal ones: Teenagers are overloaded, strapped for time, and often asked to wake far earlier than they should because of school start times. It's no surprise they're sleep-deprived as a result, with far-reaching consequences.

They're dragging themselves through their days, which begin far too early and don't end until late in the evening. And then the alarm rings at the crack of dawn and they do it all over again.

★ ★ ★

This issue hit my radar when my son entered high school in the fall of 2015. As he struggled to wake up each morning to get to class by 7:30 a.m. and came home exhausted every afternoon, I questioned why his school began classes so early. The local middle schools started at 8:45 a.m., making the transition to high school that much more difficult.

In my small community in Southern California's Inland Empire, where many residents had grown up locally and attended the same high school, no one I spoke to could remember a time when the school day *hadn't* started so early. Some thought it might be because of the buses the district had once used to transport kids, even though high school bus service had been discontinued.

It made no sense.

When I questioned parents of older kids, they shrugged and acknowledged they were grateful that stage was behind them. But it was apparent some kids were quietly suffering. My son's freshman year, there was a suicide cluster in the district.

Meanwhile, on a daily basis, kids were struggling to stay awake and get to school on time. I saw them lining up every morning at the just-opened Starbucks across the street from the school, and I talked to other parents and found out their kids were racking up tardies or quietly pursuing other options like taking online classes to avoid having a first period.

I quickly realized I'd tapped into something larger than our school or our community. In August 2015, the same month my son started high school, the CDC had released its national school-start-time survey results showing that more than three-fourths of the nation's middle and high schools started earlier than the recommended 8:30 a.m. start time.

My search for information led me to other parents in communities across the country and to findings dating back several decades. As I spoke with and met dozens of researchers, educators, and community members, it became apparent that the issue was reaching a critical mass. After many years of careful study, the American Academy of Pediatrics had issued its landmark recommendation in 2014 that middle and high schools shouldn't start before 8:30 a.m., given the relationship between too-early start times and teen sleep deprivation and the attendant risks. The CDC concurred with this recommendation when it issued the results of its school-start-time survey in 2015. Not long after, both the American Medical Association and American Psychological Association announced their support as well.

Not only was there a history dating back to the late 1990s of schools around the country that had made the change, there was a body of research documenting a track record of success: When schools shifted to later start times, students got more sleep, performed better, and were even more likely to graduate. But, despite the official health recommendations and the supporting evidence, in far too many cases, parents like me were being shut down when they tried to raise the issue.

Countless communities were like my own, unwilling to change their legacy schedules despite the overwhelming evidence.

As a journalist focused on parenting, education, and public health, I realized I'd found my new subject.

In September 2016, the *Los Angeles Times* published an op-ed I'd written about why schools should start later in the morning. The op-ed not only generated enough responses for the paper to run them the following weekend, it also caught the attention of California State Senator Anthony Portantino, who had a high schooler of his own. In early 2017, he introduced a bill requiring healthy start times for California's middle and high schools. I was quickly swept up in the legislative journey, a multi-year process that led to the first law of its kind in the country. (For more information, see Chapter 15.)

I toggled between my new role as an advocate and my background as a journalist, tracing the story not just to the very first high school to enact later start times, but even further back, to the initial research into teen sleep. And I found it all led back to a very unusual camp that had once existed, the Stanford Summer Sleep Camp.

★ ✦ ✦

The more knowledge I gained, the more I was able to implement changes to help my teens with their sleep (as well as improve my own sleep).

In these pages, I've distilled down what I learned, culled from interviews with more than fifty researchers and other experts and from close to two hundred studies, reports, books, and other sources.

I've organized the content into three main sections:

Part I provides the background and context about sleep and its increased importance during the teen years. You'll learn the story behind the Stanford Summer Sleep Camp and other key developments, as well as the reasons why schools have such early start times.

Part II delves into how our teens' sleep affects so many critical aspects of their lives, including mental health, risky behaviors, school performance, sports, driving, and more. There's also information about sleep disparities and how sex and gender, sexual identity, socioeconomic status, and race and ethnicity factor in.

Part III focuses on strategies and practical advice for improving your teen's sleep. You'll find recommendations you can implement at home, as well as resources and inspiration for changing school start times. Plus, there's an insider's view of what it took to make the California school start times law a reality, as well as an entire chapter on technology use and sleep.

★ ✦ ✹

While I was writing this book, the pandemic hit, upending life across the globe and abruptly forcing schools to pivot to online learning. Amid all of the disruption there was, for many teens, an unexpected silver lining: a chance to sleep in. Not only was their commute to school eliminated, the first class of the day was often pushed back, allowing teens to set their alarms accordingly.

It became abundantly clear schools *could* make the change, and could do so quickly. And it was apparent that in our new changed reality, our teens needed, more than ever, the emotional resilience sleep helps provide.

Some schools kept these later start times even when in-person school resumed, providing teens with the more-sleep-friendly schedules they'd needed all along. And now, with California's new law on the cusp of implementation, more than three million teens and preteens in the state will have these schedules too. As of July 1, 2022, the state's public high schools will start no earlier than 8:30 a.m., and middle schools no earlier than 8:00 a.m. (See Chapter 15 for all the details.)

★ ✦ ★

It isn't that our teens can't get by on too-little sleep—somehow, they do it when they have to, as we all do. But there are significant repercussions, as noted earlier (and which you'll learn more about in this book).

On the flip side, well-rested teens are happier and healthier and do better in school. They're more emotionally resilient. And they're easier to live with!

We *all* function better when we're not sleep-deprived.

As Dr. Rafael Pelayo, a clinical professor at Stanford University's School of Medicine who specializes in treating sleep disorders, summed up in a recent TEDx talk, "Sleeping is the most powerful and natural form of self-care we have."[5]

I hope this book gives you the information and the tools to help your teen attain more (and better) sleep. You may find it spurs you to reexamine your own sleep habits as well.

May the following pages be a road map for the journey.

PART I

. . . .

THE STORY
OF TEEN SLEEP
(AND SCHOOLS)

PROLOGUE

The Stanford Summer Sleep Camp

At the time of the Stanford Summer Sleep Camp, Lake Lagunita was still an actual lake. In the warmer months, the lake—a reservoir, technically, created by Leland Stanford in the 1870s to irrigate crops—was often a magnet for sunbathing or splashing around. It was located just behind the campers' dorm, but it was off limits for them because of their electrodes.

Joe Oliveira, one of the original campers, recalls that right after check-in, four electrodes were glued to his hair, two taped next to his eyes, and several more by his chin. The electrodes remained in place the whole time. "They had these long cords that came out of them—very small, like for an iPhone charger," he told me. During the day, the cords were often tied back and taped together into a compact bundle at the back of his head.

The "trodes" (as the campers became known because of their electrode ponytails) attracted their fair share of weird looks on their outings around the campus. Anyone observing them would have also noticed something else peculiar: like clockwork, every two hours, they all returned to the dorm for "nap tests."

In their completely darkened rooms in the dorm, all the campers—a mix of kids and teens—would lie quietly for twenty minutes and attempt to fall asleep. The entire time, technicians in a nearby control room monitored their brain waves, eye movements, and chin-muscle activity being transmitted from their electrodes via the cords, which had been plugged into a box near the headboard that had cables linked to a polysomnograph machine in the other room. There, a continuous paper trail issued forth, the jagged pattern mapping the campers' data.

When the time was up, the campers were roused and unplugged. The counselors recorded their vital signs, then plugged their wires into a second box, this one closer to the dorm room desk, and ran the campers through a short series of tests designed to measure their recall, attention span, and other aspects of alertness and cognitive functioning so these could also be assessed in relation to sleepiness. Tom Harvey, who worked as a counselor/technician at the camp for several years, recalled a mix of "math tests and memory tests and 'can you suffer through boredom' tests."

Oliveira remembered the tests more fondly. An example of a typical memory test was being asked to listen to a story about, say, a gorilla, he explained, where "gorilla" and "because" are the key words: "If you hear the word 'gorilla' you tap the left switch and when you hear the word 'because' you tap the right switch, and they want you to tap it as closely as possible to when you heard the word." Then the campers would be unplugged from the machines, their electrodes again tied back into ponytails until it was time for the next nap.

Oliveira wasn't just a camper, of course. And the Stanford Summer Sleep Camp wasn't really a camp, even though it was designed to resemble one. The campers were paid subjects for a long-term adolescent study. Each camper was paired with a counselor, who was (in nearly all cases) a Stanford undergrad working under the supervision of Mary Carskadon, who was pursuing her doctorate in neuro- and biobehavioral sciences at Stanford.

What she found, over the course of the camp's ten-year existence, profoundly changed our understanding of teen sleep.

★ ★ ★

Carskadon had arrived at Stanford a few years prior to work with William Dement, who in 1970 had founded the nation's first clinic dedicated to sleep disorders. (Dr. Dement's influence in sleep science dated back to his own days as a graduate student in the 1950s, as we'll see in the following chapter.)

In 1975, she and Dement had what he later called a lightbulb moment: as they reviewed the results of several sleep experiments, they realized the amount of time it had taken their subjects to fall asleep was directly related to how sleepy they were. This meant that measuring the amount of time it took them to fall asleep was a way to measure their level of sleepiness.

As Dement explained in his 1999 book *The Promise of Sleep*: "This may not seem like an earthshaking epiphany, but conceiving and developing an objective measure of sleepiness was perhaps one of the most important advances in sleep science."[6]

Based on this realization, they created what they called the Multiple Sleep Latency Test (MSLT) to measure how long it takes to fall asleep, which is known as sleep latency. They decided the test should be repeated every two hours. To minimize boredom (and, presumably, to keep people coming back), they decided to cap the amount of time the subjects needed to lie in bed at twenty minutes.

The common assumption was kids needed less sleep as they matured.

When the clinic received a grant to study sleep in children and teens, an opportunity presented itself for them to deploy the new MSLT measure more broadly. Their goal: to determine how sleep changed over the course of adolescence, based on the common assumption kids needed less sleep as they matured. ("This was axiomatic: the older you are, the less sleep you need," Carskadon later wrote about their pre-sleep-camp mindset.)[7]

Sleep had primarily been studied at night up until then, with far less attention paid to the impact of being sleepy during the day. "We knew we had to study the kids in the summer if we wanted to get a good full picture of their nighttime and daytime [sleep]," Carskadon told me.

But Dement's on-campus lab was too small for a study of the scope they envisioned. They needed to find a new location better suited for conducting the every-two-hour assessments. They settled on the Lambda Nu dorm, near the lake, and began to prepare.

Kim Harvey, one of Carskadon's main assistants during the camp (and sister to Tom Harvey), recalled visiting a local elementary school, now shuttered, to talk to the fifth-graders about the study and encourage them to sign up. There were also participants like Oliveira—children of Stanford faculty members who in many cases already knew the researchers. Oliveira was close friends with Dement's son and spent countless hours at their house when he was growing up.

When he and I spoke, Oliveira recounted one early adventure in which Dement wanted to see if it was possible for kids to stay up all night, in preparation for future studies about the effects of sleep deprivation on sleep latency: "We must have been ten years old. And [Dement said], 'I want to do this fun weekend. We'll be at our house the entire time . . . but we're not going to go to sleep at all. Do you think you can do that?' And of course we said, 'Heck yes!'

"We tried to go as long as we could, and we made it to the sun coming up . . . then he kept on trying to wake us up, which became highly annoying."

★ ✦ ✱

Before the campers arrived each summer, Carskadon and her crew of undergraduate assistants first had to transform Lambda Nu, with its secluded setting and corridors of empty dorm rooms, into their field lab. "It was quite a production," Carskadon recalled.

Using Dement's pickup truck, her crew of undergraduate assistants drove all over campus fetching the equipment they'd need. The sleep disorders clinic needed its polysomnograph machine year round, but there was one in the animal lab that wasn't used in the summer months, and several others tucked away at other research labs on campus. After they'd piled them all in the bed of the pickup truck to transport them to Lambda Nu, the assistants would help lug them into the building. The stainless-steel machines were large and bulky—each one nearly as tall as a refrigerator. And there were stacks of boxes of continuous feed paper for the machines—enough to fill a walk-in closet.

While the machines were being installed in the control room, several rooms in the same dorm wing were being readied for the campers. First, the windows had to be completely covered to keep any light from seeping in during the many daytime naps. In the earlier years, this was more of a hassle: each window had to be meticulously covered with cardboard, which was then duct-taped to the frames. (After a few years, the crew switched to contact paper.) Then came the task of hooking up all of the monitoring equipment, with cables snaking from the bedside and deskside consoles out the door and into the nearby control room.

And there was another challenge: after being plugged in to the bedside consoles, the campers were effectively tethered to their beds. In the absence of video monitors, intercoms, or other now-standard monitoring devices, one of Carskadon's technicians designed and built a call-button system. "For the camper, in the middle of the night, if they needed to get up to use the toilet or something, they would push a button and it would flash a light and ring a little tone in the room where the equipment was," Carskadon explained. A staff member would then go see what the camper needed. "It was old-school," she said, "but it worked really well for us."

And with that, the dorm having been converted into a sleep lab, the first wave of campers arrived for the camp's inaugural summer in 1976.

CAMP LIFE AND PROCESS

From the start, Carskadon knew the studies needed to be balanced with fun activities so campers like Oliveira would enjoy themselves and, most importantly, keep coming back. That meant volleyball games out back near the shores of the lake and afternoon strolls to Stanford's now-defunct bowling alley in the student union center.

Being out in the sun and getting sweaty meant the electrodes had to be checked regularly to ensure they hadn't come loose—if so, the area would need to be rubbed clean with alcohol before the sensors were reaffixed.

Swimming was out of the question, of course. And while the younger campers were content to go without bathing, some of the teenage campers yearned for a shower. If they decided to forgo afternoon bowling and use the time for showering, their counselor had to remove the electrodes beforehand and then reapply them post-shower. "It had to be coordinated—it wasn't a casual thing," Tom Harvey said.

At night, there were movies: reel-to-reel screenings of films borrowed from Stanford's archive during the camp's early years, and later, movies shown on a new gadget that was just becoming popular: a video cassette recorder. "Mary [Carskadon] had the first VCR I ever saw," Tom Harvey told me.

Perhaps the real draw, though, was the one-on-one attention each kid got from their counselor, whose entire role was to focus on that particular camper. "They got all that attention from this college student, which I think they really liked," Kim Harvey said.

And in fact, making the experience fun for the campers was a key part of the job. Carskadon, ever on the lookout for kids who seemed shy or unhappy, might point someone out and ask the counselors to lavish a specific camper with a little more attention, Tom Harvey recalled. Or if the kids' energy was flagging, she might ask two counselors to stage a Jell-O-eating contest as lunchtime entertainment. With the frequent naps and tests occupying so much of the day, the goal was to make the remaining pockets of time as enjoyable as possible.

At scheduled intervals throughout the day, the counselors also had to remember to administer questionnaires to assess how tired the campers felt. "Screwing up put holes in the data," Tom Harvey said. "You couldn't go back and say, 'Fill this in—we forgot to do that before.' It made a lot of statistical extra work for [Mary] when people would miss questionnaires."

Each day began with Carskadon counting down until the exact time for the counselors, clipboards in hand, to enter the kids' rooms to rouse them and record their temperature and pulse. After a quick series of tests and a questionnaire, it was time for breakfast, then back to the rooms for a morning nap period. Again, they'd be plugged in to the headboard monitors while the technicians in the control room observed their brain wave patterns for the next twenty minutes. If the kids fell asleep, the counselors would quickly reappear to wake them. And if not, the campers would lie in the darkened room until the twenty minutes were up and the counselors reappeared to untether them from their headboards.

"You had to watch them like a hawk," Kim Harvey said. "You didn't want to let the kids get sleep, because it affected the data." Using the MSLT, the technicians were measuring how long it took the kids to fall asleep (if indeed they did). But the kids weren't actually allowed to sleep until it was time for bed at night: if they'd taken even a catnap, it would have affected how sleepy they were and how long it took them to fall asleep at the next scheduled nap period. (Resting, or quiet wakefulness, was not considered to impact actual sleep.)

Then there was the matter of sleep deprivation for the staff: while the kids slept at night, they were being monitored by technicians working the night shift. "Somebody had to be missing their sleep to do the sleep research," Kim Harvey pointed out.

Perhaps the most chronically sleep-deprived was Carskadon herself, who was up each morning before the kids were awakened and stayed up late at night analyzing the polysomnograph records and noting where the various markers of sleep occurred. The late afternoon, when the kids headed off to the bowling alley, was her window for a nap.

Back then, scoring the records was all done by hand. "The machines would make little squiggly lines on a polygraph to record your brain waves and your muscle movement and your eye movement," Kim Harvey told me. "You could then score them and say, 'This is REM sleep,' 'This is non-REM sleep,' 'This is awake,' that type of thing."

For ten years, Carskadon had a cycle. At the conclusion of the camp each summer, she carted the boxes of printouts back to her lab to continue scoring all of the data—a process that would last through the fall quarter. "I would spend hours and hours and *hours* scoring the sleep records," Carskadon said. During the winter quarter, the process for the next summer's camp session would commence, with Carskadon—at the time a teaching assistant in Dement's Sleep and Dreams class—identifying promising students who could be recruited and trained as camp technicians. In the spring, she led a course to teach them the technical aspects of the role, including hooking up the electrodes and monitoring the polygraph machines. And at the conclusion of the spring quarter, as soon as that year's Lambda Nu residents had packed up and moved out, Carskadon and her crew would descend on the dorm to transform it into the Stanford Summer Sleep Camp for another summer.

★ ✦ ✦

To test the hypothesis that kids needed less sleep as they matured, Carskadon needed the same kids to come back year after year. This meant calling all of the campers ahead of time to ensure they were still planning on attending, including finding out if they had someone to drive them and even fetching them in person if necessary. The goal, Tom Harvey told me, was to ensure "no kid had a reason not to show up."

The counselors also reminded the campers to stick to a regular sleep schedule the week leading up to camp so they'd arrive well rested. They were asked to sleep ten hours a night, the same as they'd be doing at the camp, when they'd be put to bed at 10:00 p.m. and awakened at 8:00 a.m.

Up until that point, most sleep studies had been done in the context of participants' own regular sleep schedules rather than ensuring they received a fixed, optimal amount of sleep each night. Carskadon's study was one of the first to study sleep not just at night, but during the day as well, assessing the effects of nighttime sleep on daytime alertness and behavior.

Older kids didn't need less sleep: they needed the same amount, or perhaps even more.

Tracking changes in sleep as the kids matured meant assessing each child's physical development to see where they were on the puberty spectrum. Accordingly, the check-in process each summer included a brief medical exam in which fellows in Stanford's adolescent medicine program evaluated the kids using the widely accepted Tanner scale (commonly used in yearly well-child and well-adolescent pediatric checkups). A child who didn't yet show signs of puberty and was still in preadolescence was at stage one; those who showed advanced pubertal development were at stage five.

What Carskadon found, which contradicted what she'd expected, was that the kids didn't need less sleep as they matured; they needed the same amount, or perhaps even more. Across the board, all of the kids slept about nine and a quarter hours at night.

The kids who didn't yet show signs of puberty or were at the early stages would sometimes wake on their own before the counselors came in at 8:00 a.m. During the many nap times, they'd only rarely be able to fall asleep. And when they did, it took them close to ten minutes.

For the kids who were in the middle or later stages of puberty, it was a different story. In the morning, many of them had to be roused at 8:00 a.m. And at nap times, they fell asleep more often and much more quickly—in less than a minute, in some cases. (And this was after having been in bed for ten hours at night!)

Teens seemed to need more sleep than they were getting.

Carskadon and Dement didn't yet know why the more physically mature kids and teens were sleepier than the preteens, but it was obvious even then that the teens seemed to need more sleep than they were getting.

Equally intriguing but not yet fully understood, the more mature adolescents seemed to have a burst of energy in the evening, and seemed more alert (and less likely to fall asleep) during the evening nap periods. As Dement later wrote, "Mary and I cautiously attributed the results to some sort of circadian rhythm effect, but we really didn't understand them."

POST-CAMP RESEARCH

Stanford's Lambda Nu dorm is now known as the Jerry House—the result of a student-led effort to rename it in honor of Jerry Garcia of the Grateful Dead. A sprawling lounge with a two-story row of windows runs along the rear of the building, providing an expansive view of the meadow of wheat-colored grass filling the now-dry lake bed and the native oaks just beyond it.

At the entrance to the lounge, mostly unnoticed by the undergrads who pass through, is a glass-and-wood plaque commemorating the camp: "Stanford University Summer Sleep Camp, 1976–1985. May All Who Live in This House Have Refreshing Sleep and Pleasant Dreams."

In 2012, when the plaque was unveiled during a reunion event, Carskadon flew back to attend. She's at Brown University now, where she's the director of chronobiology and sleep research at Bradley Hospital (part of the medical school at Brown University). She also heads the Sleep for Science Research Lab, where she established the next iteration of sleep camp and continued her groundbreaking research into adolescent sleep.

In one such study, Carskadon surveyed several hundred sixth-graders as a way to examine the circadian timing shift she and Dement had earlier surmised. One set of questions allowed researchers to assess the students' stage of physical maturity, and another series of questions revealed whether they felt most alert in the morning or in the evening. The results were striking: girls in the earlier stages of puberty tended to keep earlier hours, while those who were further along in their pubertal development were far more likely to report keeping later hours. (The change in boys was much slighter, given that their pubertal development lagged behind the girls.)[8]

Numerous subsequent in-lab studies at Brown allowed Carskadon to test this more directly. By analyzing levels of melatonin, the hormone that encourages sleep, via saliva samples taken at regular intervals, she was able to show that adolescents indeed undergo a shift during the teen years: compared to younger kids, their melatonin levels rise later at night and don't subside until later in the morning.

As Carskadon discovered, this shift in teens' internal body clocks explains why they're not able to fall asleep until later in the evening and why they tend to sleep in whenever possible.

During the Stanford camp's ten-year run, Carskadon also studied sleep disorders like narcolepsy and sleep apnea and analyzed how sleep patterns change in the elderly. At Brown, she continues to run studies on both kids and adults on a variety of sleep-related topics, including ADHD and sleep and the effects of alcohol on sleep.

As Carskadon discovered, the shift in teens' internal body clocks explains why they're not able to fall asleep until later in the evening.

But all of this knowledge came later. As Kim Harvey told me, recalling her time working at the Stanford Summer Sleep Camp, "We hardly knew anything about sleep back then."

CHAPTER 1

Sleep and the Teenage Brain: Why Sleep Is So Important, Especially During Adolescence

When my son was a toddler, every morning began the same way. "Come in!" he'd shout at 6:30 a.m., hollering to my husband and me to free him from his crib. It was better than it had been—as a baby, my son woke several times each night and napped only fitfully. Nevertheless, I was relieved when those sleep-deprived years finally ended and assumed sleep issues were behind us.

Enter the teen years. Suddenly, the child who used to wake early and happily was moody and hard to rouse in the mornings. By the time he started his freshman year of high school in August 2015, it was obvious he'd reached a new phase where his body clock was painfully out of sync with the rhythms of daily life. As I drove him to school each morning in time for the 7:30 a.m. start, all I had to do was look over at him to see he was barely awake, much less ready to learn.

His struggles to wake up early weren't unique, of course. He'd merely morphed into a teenager. Amid everything else about him that was changing, his sleep needs were too. In fact, not only was his sleep timing shifting, his sleep was more important than it had been since his babyhood.

As we'll cover in this chapter, the sleep our kids get during the teen years plays a critical role in their development.

Before we get to that, though, let's take a step back to review the basics about sleep—including why we do it.

WHAT SLEEP IS—AND WHAT IT ISN'T

Although we spend a whopping one-third of our lives asleep, very little was known about it until relatively recently.

As recently as about two hundred years ago, Scottish physician Robert Macnish defined sleep as the intermediate state between wakefulness and death.

The prevailing belief was that our brains basically shut down when we slumbered, which made sleep research seem rather dull. "No one bothered to study it because it was defined by what it wasn't," Elizabeth Kolbert wrote in the *New Yorker*. "Sleep was a state of not being awake and, at the same time, of not being comatose or dead."[9]

This mindset endured until about a century ago, when Nathaniel Kleitman created the world's first permanent sleep lab at the University of Chicago. Using a vacant two-room chemistry laboratory, he turned one room into a bedroom, furnished with a cot, and the other into an observation post.

Then, in the 1950s, Kleitman dispatched one of his graduate students, Eugene Aserinsky, to local homes to observe babies as they napped. There, he noticed the sleeping infants had predictable patterns when their eyeballs were moving under their eyelids.[10]

Kleitman and Aserinsky were intrigued and wanted to find out if sleeping adults had the same eye movements. But rather than hovering nearby to keep watch all night long, they came up with a less tedious method. As Dement recounted in *The Promise of Sleep*, electrodes affixed near the person's eyes recorded and transmitted their eye movements, which were then printed out in a long, continuous pattern depicting when the eyes were moving and when they were still.[11]

Aserinsky noticed there were times when the printing pens suddenly zigzagged across the paper. It wasn't a printer malfunction, as he first surmised: the jerky movements were recording what he and Kleitman decided to call "rapid eye movement" (REM).

Dement—who would go on to found the sleep lab at Stanford in 1970—was at that point a medical student at the University of Chicago working in the lab with them. After numerous all-night recordings documenting the new phenomenon, Dement realized these periods of rapid eye movement occurred in predictable cycles. He divided them into four non-REM stages and a fifth state of REM. "At the time, I made up those names casually," Dement wrote in 1999. "Simply making up the names for sleep stages is something I would never have the audacity to do now."[12]

Stages of Sleep

At night, the brain cycles through a series of distinct stages, as first identified by Dement:

Stage one—Transition: This is the lightest (and briefest) stage, when we drift off to sleep. Our bodies sometimes twitch or jerk as we're falling asleep, and we can be startled awake by even a minor noise.

Stage two—Light sleep: As our breathing and heart rate continue to slow, we enter stage two, a cycle of light sleep that makes up about half of our overall time asleep.

Stage three—Deep sleep: This stage of sleep is the deepest and the most difficult to wake from. (What Dement had initially called stages three and four of non-REM sleep have since been consolidated into this stage.)[13]

REM sleep: The final stage, REM, is when most dreams occur. Although our eyes are moving rapidly, our bodies are temporarily immobilized, which is what keeps us from acting out our dreams (although there is a rare disorder in which this can happen).[14]

Stages one through three are all considered non-REM sleep. We continue to cycle through these stages throughout the night, but the balance shifts: during the first third of the night, we sleep more deeply (spending more time in stage three non-REM sleep), but as the night wears on, the dreaming phase, REM sleep, gradually lengthens. In fact, about three-fourths of REM sleep takes place during the second half of the night.[15]

WHAT HAPPENS WHEN WE SLEEP?

The discovery of REM sleep in 1952 and the ability to record brain and eye movements throughout the night showed that sleep isn't the equivalent of powering down. Instead, it's actually when our brains sort through and process all the information and stimuli we've taken in during the day, with each sleep stage having a distinct function.

From babies learning to walk to pianists perfecting a difficult piece, lighter non-REM sleep (stage two) plays a critical role, Matthew Walker, a neuroscientist at the University of California, Berkeley, wrote in *Why We Sleep*.[16] The parts of the brain responsible for learning and refining these tasks show increased brain activity the night after these actions, he noted.[17]

When it comes to learning and retaining information, such as studying for a test or memorizing vocabulary words, deep non-REM sleep (stage three) becomes key. New knowledge is first saved in short-term storage, in what Walker terms the "temporary warehouse" of the hippocampus. During deep non-REM sleep, the information moves to its long-term home in the cortex to free up the brain's short-term storage for new input.[18] This process is akin to "clearing out the cache of short-term memory for the new imprinting of facts, while accumulating an ever-updated catalog of past memories," Walker wrote.[19]

This stage three deep sleep is also when we reflect on what we've learned, in effect analyzing the newly acquired information as it's prepared for storage, he noted.[20] Then, during REM sleep, our brains integrate this information with our past experiences, blending it together to forge new insights.

Our nightly REM sleep is also what makes us more creative and insightful, as it's when our brains assess the various bits of information we've gathered during the day to weave them together into something more lasting.

This can lead to a breakthrough on a vexing problem, or to a new inspiration entirely. In fact, the blockbuster *Twilight* series first came to author Stephenie Meyer in a dream. One morning, she woke from a particularly vivid dream about a girl and a sparkly vampire who were falling in love. "I stayed in bed, thinking about the dream. I was so intrigued by the nameless couple's story that I hated the idea of forgetting it," Meyer recounted. Instead, she got up and began to write.[21]

Nighttime is also a time of healing and of growth, spurred by the growth hormone the pituitary gland releases while we're sleeping. This hormone doesn't just trigger growth for babies through young adults; it also activates the body's ability to heal from injuries.[22]

Sleep even helps regulate appetite, keeping the two hormones that control feelings of hunger in proper balance.[23]

RECOMMENDED SLEEP BY AGE

In 2015, after synthesizing the results of more than three hundred studies published during the previous decade, the National Sleep Foundation released updated guidelines for recommended sleep by age group. In most cases this broadened the ranges: for teens, for example, the new range is eight to ten hours per night, compared to eight-and-a-half to nine-and-a-half hours previously.[24] (That said, it's important to point out that eight hours is the *minimum* recommended amount; while this may suffice for some teens, others will need closer to ten.)

Unfortunately, there's a huge gap between the recommendations and reality. In 2018, a report released by the CDC noted that 43 percent of high schoolers were averaging six or fewer hours of sleep per night![25]

	Age Range	Recommended Hours of Sleep
Newborn	0–3 months old	14–17 hours
Infant	4–11 months old	12–15 hours
Toddler	1–2 years old	11–14 hours
Preschool	3–5 years old	10–13 hours
School-age	6–13 years old	9–11 hours
Teen	14–17 years old	8–10 hours
Young adult	18–25 years old	7–9 hours
Adult	26–64 years old	7–9 hours
Older adult	65 or more years old	7–8 hours

Source: National Sleep Foundation

A Quick Look at Brain Development

Babies are born with far more neural cells than they'll ultimately need. This primes them to be able to absorb all the sights, sounds, and other stimuli to come, as neuroscientist Frances Jensen noted in *The Teenage Brain*.[26]

For example, infants' brains are broadly attuned to the sounds of many different languages, Adriana Galván, who directs the Developmental Neuroscience Laboratory at the University of California, Los Angeles, told me. But this capability falls away as children learn the language (or languages) around them. "It wouldn't make sense for the brain to hold on to this malleability for all languages of the world," she explained, "because it would preclude becoming experts in our own language."

During the process of learning, the synapses connecting the neurons increase and become stronger. "In the first few years of childhood, there is a critical period of plasticity in which learning comes quickly and easily," Jensen has written.[27]

There's a second major phase of brain development still to come, however, during adolescence. This time, the focus is on pruning and remodeling the initial structure.[28]

The neurons being used the most develop the strongest connections, or synapses, between them, while those that aren't being used (the surplus created during the initial phase) are removed. Getting rid of this neural deadwood helps the remaining neurons work more efficiently. (The term "use it or lose it" really is true when it comes to teens' brain cells!) This pruning takes place during stage three (deep sleep).[29]

Even as this pruning is taking place, teen brains are enhancing the connections between neurons through a process called myelination (referring to myelin, the white matter in the brain). Myelin, a fatty substance, is what insulates the neural connections and allows the signals to travel more quickly—a process Galván likens to upgrading a dirt road to a paved freeway. There's also a strengthening of connections *between* areas of the brain that takes place during adolescence, she explained. These enhancements affect how quickly teen brains process information. However, poor-quality sleep may slow the maturation of the connectivity process.[30]

SLEEP QUALITY

How long you sleep matters, but so does how *well* you sleep.

"Sleep quality, we've found, is just as important, if not more so, than sleep quantity," Galván said. "When you're getting disrupted sleep or low-quality sleep, you're not getting the restorative benefits."

She explained, "You may be in bed for nine hours, but if you're woken up in what are called micro-awakenings and you don't even realize that you're waking up, that's going to disrupt your sleep—or at the very least, make you not feel rested in the morning."

And of course, the awakenings you *are* aware of—those middle-of-the-night episodes where it feels like you're just staring at the ceiling—erode both actual sleep time and the perceived quality of that sleep.

In a recent study of more than a thousand young adults in New Zealand and the United States, researchers found sleep quality mattered more than diet, exercise, or even amount of sleep as a predictor of mental health and well-being. (Sleep quality was assessed by asking participants to rate how refreshed they felt upon waking.)[31]

Similar findings were reported in a 2020 study of more than four thousand college students: those who said they got "restful sleep" at least four nights a week were less likely to report depressive symptoms (and had higher grade point averages).[32]

For a more detailed look at sleep and mental health, see Chapter 4.

THE TIMING OF TEEN SLEEP

The explanation for why teens don't get enough sleep goes back to their biological clocks. As Carskadon found, during puberty, melatonin, the hormone that primes the body for sleep, is released later in the evening and doesn't subside until later in the morning.

Teen sleep shifts accordingly. Until the melatonin kicks in late at night, teens don't start feeling sleepy. And until it recedes (later in the morning than it used to), it's harder for teens to rouse themselves out of bed.[33] "The students may be in school," Carskadon has written, "but their brains are at home on their pillows."[34]

You'd think perpetually sleepy teenagers would want to fall asleep earlier, but that's not the case.

In general, the longer we're awake, the sleepier we get. This is referred to as sleep pressure, and it takes longer to build up in teens than in younger kids.[35] But there are still times of the day when we're more alert (despite having been up for several hours) due to our biological clock. This internal timing is what signals us to wake and feel alert in the day, and it also provides a second boost in the evening to help us power through the remaining hours before we're finally sleepy enough for bed.

In teens, the entire process shifts later. Not only do their melatonin levels not subside until later in the morning, their second wave of alertness comes later in the evening as well. As a parent, you may be ready to start winding down for the night, but due to this "troublesome kick in alertness,"[36] as Dement characterized it, your teen won't start feeling that way until about 11:00 p.m.[37]

AN IMPORTANT NOTE ABOUT PUBERTY

When it comes to puberty, not all kids are on the same timetable. Girls start the process earlier, anywhere between ages eight and thirteen, while boys are about a year behind.[38] We've all seen the visible differences: some girls are already towering over the boys by sixth grade and starting to appear more physically mature, while their male classmates still look like kids. This doesn't just make for awkward pairings at school dances; it also has important implications for girls' sleep.

In her study of sixth-graders, Carskadon found that kids who were already in the midst of puberty generally reported having later bedtimes than their peers. (This was the case for the majority of the girls but fewer of the boys, who were less likely to have started puberty.)[39] In later studies, she found an association between puberty and the later release of melatonin: kids who were further along in their physical development had already shifted to the later melatonin timing (driving the later sleep pattern).[40]

Even as girls[41] and boys[42] now start puberty younger than they used to—which cues them to stay up later at night and sleep in later in the morning—school start times have actually shifted *earlier*. (More on this is in Chapter 2.)

WHAT HAPPENS WHEN TEENS' ALARM CLOCKS GO OFF IN THE MORNING

For starters, they're probably groggy, especially if they're being forced to wake up well before they've achieved the recommended amount of sleep. For teens, as previously noted, that's eight to ten hours.

This abrupt waking also cuts into their REM sleep, which is back-loaded so more of it happens during the second half of the night. This means they get less of the sleep stage that fuels their creativity, helps them synthesize information, and even helps regulate their emotions. (In an analysis of the results of the national Youth Risk Behavior Survey, researchers found that as teens' sleep went down, their odds of engaging in risky behaviors went up, ranging from drinking alcohol to carrying a weapon to considering or even attempting suicide.)[43]

We'll look at these various behaviors in more depth in later chapters.

WHY SCHOOL START TIMES MATTER

Given that adolescents can't fall asleep until later in the evening, they'd need to be able to wake up at a correspondingly later time to attain the recommended eight to ten hours of sleep. *But this can't happen if they have to be at school early in the morning.*

Consider what a too-early start time does to teen sleep: if our teenagers can't fall asleep until about 11:00 p.m., getting eight hours of sleep means not having to wake until 7:00 a.m. the next morning. That's just to achieve the low end of the recommended eight to ten hours, and this also assumes teens actually fall asleep right when they go to bed.

Unlike internal body clocks, however, school start times *can* be changed as a way to help teens get more sleep. Since 2014, when the American

Academy of Pediatrics issued its landmark recommendation that middle and high schools should start at 8:30 a.m. or later,[44] the consensus for this approach (along with the research demonstrating the link between later start times and teen sleep) has continued to grow, as we'll see in the following chapters.

A Note about Daylight

Especially in winter, it's dark when kids are getting up and it's *still* dark when they arrive at school. Lacking daylight to help cue their brains that it's time to be alert, these students often have to force themselves to get out of bed, and then struggle to stay awake in their first classes of the day. (Imagine getting to work in the dark and trying to feel energetic and productive.)

In cities at more northern latitudes, this is even more pronounced. In Minneapolis in December, for example, the sun doesn't even rise until after 7:30 a.m. (although the sky gradually starts to lighten before then).[45]

TEEN-SLEEP TAKEAWAYS

- We cycle through four stages of sleep each night, with each having a distinct function.

- The teen years are a critical period for brain development.

- Teens need eight to ten hours of sleep each night.

- The timing of sleep shifts during the teen years, driven by puberty.

- Quality and quantity of sleep both matter.

- Too-early school start times are a main factor cutting into teen sleep.

CHAPTER 2

How Did We Get Here?

At this point, you may be wondering: "Why does school start so early, anyway? Has this always been the case?"

The answer is no, it wasn't always this way, and the reasons for the change have absolutely nothing to do with student well-being.

About a century ago, high schools in the western United States started at 9:00 a.m. according to a 2013 report unearthed by SchoolStartTime.org.[46] But by 2017, the average start time in the United States had shifted to 8:00 a.m., with more than 40 percent of schools starting even earlier than that. In fact, more than 10 percent of US public high schools started before 7:30 a.m., with some far earlier than that.[47]

WHEN HIGH SCHOOL WAS "A ROOM IN AN ELEMENTARY SCHOOL"

Even though the first public high school opened its doors in 1821, it took more than a century for the concept to really catch on. "Many of these early high schools were little more than a room in an elementary school," Thomas Hine wrote in *The Rise and Fall of the American Teenager*.[48] There were far more teens laboring in factories or on farms than attending high school, he noted, given that the majority of high-school-aged teens had to work to help support their families.[49]

By the end of the century, however, an average of one new high school was opening every single day.[50] High school enrollment doubled between 1900 and 1910, then quadrupled by 1920 to more than two million teens.[51] Around this timeframe, as the 1913 report notes, school started around 9:00 a.m.

(A quick note on historical start-time data: It would be easier to track the shift in start times if there were a centralized database, but unfortunately this type of resource doesn't exist. However, researchers have still been able to document the change by looking at old reports, archived schedules, and more recent surveys.)

Despite the steady growth of high schools, it wasn't until the Great Depression wiped out millions of jobs that attending high school became a more viable alternative to working. In 1920, only about 30 percent of American teens attended high school; by 1936, more than 60 percent did.[52]

Both child labor laws and New Deal federal relief programs played important roles, historian Paula Fass noted in *The End of American Childhood*.[53]

At the same time, high school was quickly becoming an entrenched part of the adolescent experience. "By the middle of the twentieth century," wrote Fass, "high school life defined and normalized adolescence."[54]

The first members of the Baby Boom generation entered high school in the early 1960s, and more and more high schools began to sprout up to accommodate them all. This included opening schools in the newly built and fast-growing suburbs.

THE COLD WAR AS CATALYST

With high school now playing a key role in preparing students for college or for going directly into the workforce, educators focused on refining the curriculum and making other improvements. As Hine noted in *The Rise and Fall of the American Teenager,* the Cold War era fueled the belief that US education (especially in the areas of math and science) lagged behind the Soviet Union, requiring urgent changes to maintain America's competitiveness.[55]

These recommended educational changes were outlined in an influential report written by retired Harvard University president James Bryant Conant in 1959. After evaluating schools around the country, Conant concluded that school size was crucial for providing a high-quality comprehensive education. Specifically, he recommended high schools have graduating class sizes of at least one hundred "to function adequately."[56] At the time, one-third of the nation's high schools didn't meet this threshold. He recommended these schools be consolidated into larger schools, which could provide a comprehensive curriculum.

Although school consolidation had already been taking place, Conant's recommendations received widespread attention and helped spur the closure of many smaller schools and the rise of larger school districts. (Even as late as 1950, there were still around 60,000 one-room schools in the United States; by 1960, the number had shrunk to about 20,000.)[57]

THE YELLOW SCHOOL BUS

Without these small local schools, typically located within walking distance of students' homes, school buses became increasingly common. By 1950, they were ferrying about seven million kids to and from school each day.[58]

The growth of suburbia was also well under way, and with it, the construction of scores of new schools in more far-flung locations. Another change: a cultural shift away from letting kids walk or bike to school, due to the perceived potential danger.[59]

By the 1970s, economic realities, including recession, inflation, higher fuel costs, and lower enrollment, created a strong pressure to cut transportation costs, as noted in a comprehensive school-start-time report released by Children's National Medical Center in 2014.[60]

Many school districts sought to minimize their costs by shifting to a tiered bus system, using the same fleet of buses for staggered runs instead of maintaining and operating separate buses for elementary, middle, and high schools.

A SHIFT TO EARLIER STARTS

This, in turn, meant adjusting school starting and ending times. The general consensus was that teens, being older, were better suited for early start times than young children. (This was before the research into adolescent sleep.) As a result, high schools were often placed in the earliest slots, followed by middle schools and elementary schools.

The effects on start times were dramatic. Even as recently as the 1950s and 1960s, high schools had generally started between 8:30 and 9:00 a.m.[61] But by the 2007–08 school year, when the National Center for Educational Statistics began tracking the data as part of its secondary school surveys, **the average start time for US public high schools had crept up to 8:04 a.m.** Moreover, close to 9 percent of schools were starting prior to 7:30 a.m.

Recently, two research economists took another look at the 2007–08 data and discovered something interesting: the start-time changes initially driven by suburbanization and consolidation had endured. Schools classified as suburban (based on US Census data) had earlier start times than urban schools, as did larger schools compared to smaller ones, the researchers noted.[62]

Also noteworthy: a study of high school schedules found that schools with early start times had shifted *even earlier* over time[63]—further proof that this early-start mindset has become more entrenched over the years.

The result: as of 2017–18, the most recent data available, the average public high school start time was 8:00 a.m.[64]

(For additional information, a great resource is the comprehensive historical timeline included in Children's National Medical Center 2014 school-start-time report.)

THE GREAT SLEEP RECESSION—AND NOT JUST FOR TEENS

As you'd expect, the shift to earlier start times corresponds with an erosion of teen sleep over the last few decades. In a report aptly titled "The Great Sleep Recession," researchers took a look at teens' reported sleep every year from 1991 to 2012, using data gathered via the longstanding Monitoring the Future survey.[65]

What they found was disturbing. Not only did teen sleep decline over time, it was markedly worse for specific groups, including girls, who were less likely than boys to get at least seven hours' sleep.

Sleep diminished during middle and high school, they found, but fifteen-year-olds had the biggest decline: in 1991, 72 percent of them said they regularly got at least seven hours of sleep per night, but by 2012, only 63 percent did. (And even seven hours of sleep is far short of the eight-to-ten-hour range recommended for teens.)

Teens aren't the only ones getting more tired. There's been a similar decline for adults, whose nightly sleep has also dwindled over time. Gallup polls show that in 1942, 84 percent of American adults reported getting at least seven hours of sleep, but by 2013, just 59 percent did. Even worse: in 2013, 40 percent of adults reported six hours of sleep or less.[66]

More recently, a 2020 poll by the National Sleep Foundation found that about half of American adults reported feeling sleepy at least three days a week, and a quarter said this "sometimes" or "often" interferes with their daily activities.

Against this backdrop, it's not surprising that a widespread understanding of the teen sleep epidemic has been slow in coming, or that legacy school start times have endured. Entrenched attitudes can be hard to dislodge.

Teen Sleep in Other Countries

Teens in the United States aren't the only ones who are sleep-deprived. Compared to their counterparts in European and Asian countries, they're roughly in the middle. A 2010 meta-analysis of studies in twenty countries over a thirty-year period found that US teens generally got less school-night sleep (by up to an hour) than European teens. But, they fared far better than teens in Asian countries, who lagged by one to two hours a night![67]

As for start times: there isn't a ready data source, but they, too, vary quite a bit, as reported by a range of sources and studies. In Australia, the norm is 8:30 to 9:00 a.m.,[68] and in Singapore, it's 7:30 a.m.[69] In the United States, the average start for public high schools is 8:00 a.m.,[70] but in Canada, it's considerably later: 8:43 a.m. for secondary schools.[71]

Where do teens get the most sleep? Flemish Belgium, according to a 2020 analysis of twenty-three European countries and Canada. Teens there averaged more than nine hours on weeknights (based on self-reported data). Other countries where teens got at least eight and a half hours of sleep included Canada, Norway, French Belgium, Wales, Denmark, and the Netherlands. Even teens in the lowest-ranked country, Poland, still averaged about seven and three-quarter hours of sleep.[72]

TEEN-SLEEP TAKEAWAYS

- Schools used to start later in the morning. As a result of consolidation, busing, and budget considerations, the morning bell gradually moved earlier.

- Teen sleep has also declined over time.

- Sleep deprivation is widespread. Many adults also regularly don't get the recommended number of hours.

- Teen sleep varies by country—it's generally better in Europe than in the United States and worse in Asia.

CHAPTER 3

Taking It to the Schools

Knowledge is one thing; change is another. Despite sleep researcher Mary Carskadon's discoveries at the Stanford Summer Sleep Camp in the 1970s and '80s, it took a while for news about the mismatch between teens' body clocks and school schedules to reach the high school campus.

That crucial step—using the knowledge of teens' circadian rhythms to adjust school start times as a way to help teens get more sleep—didn't take place until 1996, in a location far removed from Carskadon's original research in California or her subsequent move to Rhode Island's Brown University. Instead, it took place in Edina, an upscale Minneapolis suburb.

THE EDINA STORY

In 1993, Carskadon was invited to present her research about sleepiness in adolescence to the Minnesota Regional Sleep Disorders Center in Minneapolis.

Maurice Dysken, a now-retired psychiatrist who attended her presentation, was at that time the father of a teenage daughter whose school started at 7:20 a.m.—an "absurd" start time, he said, recalling how she used to wait for the school bus in the pre-dawn darkness. "You could see the stars at that hour. I thought, 'This is nuts.' "

After hearing Carskadon's talk, Dysken and Mark Mahowald, who headed the center, discussed how they could get the word out more broadly in the community. Dysken, who was president of the Minnesota Psychiatric

Society, decided to bring it to the attention of the Minnesota Medical Association. Getting the group's backing meant passing a resolution, which they did later that year. That fall, every superintendent in the state's 450 school districts received a mailing about teen sleep and the association's recommendation of later start times.

And then: nothing, as confirmed by a follow-up survey to the superintendents a year later.

This time around, though, the information caught the attention of Ken Dragseth, superintendent of the Edina School District.

As it turned out, interest in teen sleep had already been bubbling up at the district's high school. The health teacher there, Pacy Erck, had long had sleep as part of her curriculum, even bringing in a sleep technician from the local hospital to talk to the students.

There was also a newly hired Edina High School principal, Ron Tesch, and he and Erck had begun discussing the idea of later start times.

Tesch first visited Erck's classes to talk to the students about their sleep habits, then solicited feedback from the school's teachers. They were "very much aware of the comatose situation of young people in their classes, and pretty much with us from the start," he recalled.

Tesch and Erck then broached the topic with Dragseth, the superintendent.

When Dragseth received the medical association's letter recommending later start times, it was "an 'aha' moment," he told me. Not only did it dovetail with Tesch and Erck's efforts, it squared with his own experience watching tired teens struggle to stay awake in school.

Other superintendents in Edina's athletic league were less amenable, given the potential changes to their game schedules. "It was a very hostile crowd, and I'd known these people for years," Dragseth said. "This brought such intense emotions." But they, too, ultimately came around.

Then there was the issue of school buses, given that changing the drop-offs and pickups for Edina High School would have a ripple effect on the district's elementary and middle schools. The district ended up evaluating twenty-two different scenarios before selecting one that kept transportation costs the same and had minimal impact on the other schools' schedules.

Overall, it was a two-year process, including extensive outreach to parents and others who would be affected. "**A well-informed community is usually a much more supportive community**," Tesch pointed out.

And so, in the fall of 1996, after a year of preparation, Edina High School moved its start time from 7:25 a.m. to 8:30 a.m.

Dragseth had assumed others in the state—and perhaps even around the country—were taking similar steps. As it turned out, Edina was the only one.

The changes were immediate. "Within those first few weeks, especially teachers who had first-hour classes said, 'We just can't believe the difference—these kids are awake, they're alert,'" Dragseth said.

There were smaller changes too, like custodians noticing fewer discarded coffee cups and Coke cans littering the hallways.

And then there were the students themselves, like Tyler Anderson, who was a senior that year and played on the varsity football and basketball teams. "I love it," he told the *Star Tribune* in December 1996. Not only had his grades gone up, he no longer felt "like a zombie" during first period, he said.[73]

A GAME CHANGER

Beyond the anecdotal evidence, there were also more formal evaluations under way. Shortly after the Edina school board approved the time change, Dragseth had reached out to Kyla Wahlstrom, who was the associate director at the Center for Applied Research and Educational Improvement at the University of Minnesota.

"Honestly, I was so skeptical," Wahlstrom told me. Before joining the research center, Wahlstrom had spent nineteen years as a teacher, special-education director, and principal. Even as a principal, she'd always assumed teens were just naturally sleepy. "You don't even question the normalcy," she recalled.

The results from Edina were a game changer. "It was just this amazing amount of positive data," Wahlstrom said. "I heard teachers say, 'The kids are now awake in the first hour.' Counselors and nurses said that these kids were self-referring less for depression and somatic complaints. The principal said the building was calmer and there was less agitation in the hallway and in the cafeteria. And 92 percent of parents said that the kids were easier to live with."

The results quickly spread to the much-larger Minneapolis school district, which already had a multi-school consortium working with the research center. Minneapolis was more diverse and far-flung than Edina, with seven public high schools and about 51,000 students district-wide. Still, based on what Wahlstrom had found and the underlying medical research, the school board voted nearly unanimously to follow suit, shifting its high school start times from 7:15 a.m. to 8:40 a.m. in the fall of 1997.

Again, Wahlstrom was on hand. Using data collected both before and after the change, she conducted the first longitudinal study examining the impact of later school start times, looking at everything from school attendance to students' reported sleep prior to the change and three years after.

The results of that report, published in 2002, were striking: After the start-time change, students got an additional hour of sleep on school nights and were less likely to feel depressed. Attendance rates went up. And students still participated in after-school sports and other activities at the same levels, refuting a common concern about later end times.[74]

Wahlstrom's findings weren't just front-page news in Minneapolis; they also sparked widespread interest. "I did interviews with more than thirty national newspapers," she told me.

The Z's to A's Act

Around this time, US Rep. Zoe Lofgren, from San Jose, California, was struggling with getting her two kids out of bed in the morning. When her eldest hit the teen years, "All of a sudden, we couldn't get her up," Lofgren told me. She wondered, "Am I a bad mother?"

A Stanford graduate, Lofgren reached out to William Dement, director of the Stanford Sleep Medicine Clinic, to learn more. After speaking to him and Mary Carskadon and learning about teen sleep patterns, Lofgren realized it wasn't her; it was her teens' biology and the mismatch with school start times that was causing the issue.

"And I thought, 'Why would we do that?'" Lofgren said. "By starting high school later, you could accommodate the biology of these young students—teenagers—and let them get enough sleep."

Even now, Lofgren recalls the "ridiculous" timing of an extra math course her son took during high school, which met at about 6:20 a.m. "It was added on to the early morning, which was too early anyhow," she said, characterizing it as a "staggering assault on sleep."

Although Congress doesn't have jurisdiction over school start times, Lofgren set out to raise visibility for the issue. In 1998, she introduced the Z's to A's Act, which she's reintroduced five times since (most recently in 2019).[75] She's continued to advocate for later start times over the last twenty-plus years.

AMPING UP ADVOCACY

Teen sleep had also hit the radar of the CDC, which added a question about teen sleep to its 2007 national Youth Risk Behavior Survey (part of a comprehensive system of surveys the CDC conducts every two years to monitor a wide range of health behaviors). Those results, published in 2008, showed almost 70 percent of high schoolers were averaging less than eight hours of sleep on school nights.[76]

Meanwhile, like Lofgren, other parents were also noticing how difficult it was to get their teens out of bed in the morning. In Maryland, Terra Ziporyn Snider had already been advocating for later start times for a decade, to no avail, when she decided to launch an online petition in 2011. For Ziporyn Snider, coauthor of *The New Harvard Guide to Women's Health*, it was personal: the high school her three kids attended started at 7:17 a.m., and her sleep-deprived son had recently backed the car into the garage door because he'd forgotten to open it.

Not only did the petition soon amass five thousand signatures, it prompted others to reach out to her, including another local mom, Maribel Ibrahim. Together, they launched the group Start School Later to raise awareness.

"Every Wednesday, we would go to the Capitol and visit various legislators' offices, present the petition with signers from their districts, and talk to them about the issue," Ziporyn Snider told me.

The group also drew in other like-minded parents and researchers both locally and beyond. "What I really came to realize very quickly," Ziporyn Snider said, "was that there were people like me who had been doing this for years all over the country."

Previously, "the sleep researchers were talking to other sleep researchers, the educators were talking to other educators, and the advocates were working in their own little communities." Start School Later brought them under one umbrella.

"I think it was the founding of Start School Later that really jump-started more national momentum," Amy Wolfson, a psychology professor at Loyola University Maryland who serves on the group's advisory board, told me.

Even as this was happening, the research continued. In early 2014, Wahlstrom published the results of a sweeping study, funded by the CDC, examining the health and academic outcomes of later start times at eight high schools in three states. At the schools that started at 8:30 a.m. or later, the majority of students were able to get at least eight hours of sleep. Other benefits included increased on-time attendance and fewer car crashes.[77]

Meanwhile, Judith Owens, who was then director of sleep medicine at Children's National Medical Center in Washington, DC, had embarked on an ambitious analysis of school districts around the country that had already changed their start times. The study had been commissioned by nearby Fairfax County Public Schools in Virginia—one of the largest districts in the nation—where a community group had already been advocating for later start times for a decade.

Lacking a central data source of schools that had made the shift (something that *still* doesn't exist), Owens' team scoured multiple sources, then reached out to districts around the country to gather detailed information and identify best practices. The report,[78] published in 2014, received widespread coverage and has been shared with numerous other districts since then.

DOCTORS' RECOMMENDATIONS

During this same timeframe, Owens, who now directs the Center for Pediatric Sleep Disorders at Boston Children's Hospital, was also part of a working group on adolescent sleep for the American Academy of Pediatrics. **In August 2014, the group released its landmark policy statement calling for middle and high schools to start no earlier than 8:30 a.m.**[79]

"The way we framed this was that this is a health issue, this is a health and safety issue," Owens, the statement's lead author, told me. She was well aware the policy, which took five years to develop, would carry tremendous weight. As she noted in remarks released by the organization, it was "a definitive and powerful statement about the importance of sleep to the health, safety, performance and well-being of our nation's youth."

Other major groups soon followed suit, including the American Psychological Association, American Medical Association, and American Academy of Sleep Medicine.

There was an additional piece, which the CDC was able to provide: a snapshot of school start times for nearly 40,000 public secondary schools. The data, which had been obtained by the US Department of Education as part of the 2011–12 School and Staffing Survey, allowed researchers from the two organizations to compile the first comprehensive examination of middle- and high-school start times in every state.[80]

Among their findings: **nationwide, only about 18 percent of schools were meeting the "8:30 a.m. or later" guideline.** The average start time was 8:03 a.m., but there were dramatic differences at the state level. (The earliest average start time, 7:40 a.m., was in Louisiana, where about 30 percent of schools started the day before 7:30 a.m.)

Again, when the CDC released its report in 2015, the topic received widespread coverage. But more importantly, because the data had been gathered prior to the statements by the AAP and others, it would serve as an important baseline for measuring change.

TEEN-SLEEP TAKEAWAYS

- Results from the first schools to adopt later start times in the 1990s showed that students got more sleep as a result.

- Educating the community and addressing issues were both critical for success.

- Since then, the amount of research and support for later school start times has continued to grow.

- The American Academy of Pediatrics' 2014 landmark statement recommending start times of 8:30 a.m. or later prompted similar recommendations from many other major groups.

- A 2015 report by the CDC (with data gathered prior to the AAP statement) showed that just 18 percent of schools met the guideline, with an average secondary school start time of 8:03 a.m.

PART II

. . . .

WHY
SLEEP MATTERS

CHAPTER 4

Sleep and Mental Health

Taylor Ruiz Chiu was any college's dream candidate: a hard-driving honors student who played water polo, participated in theater, played trombone in three school bands, and was also a Girl Scout. And that was just freshman year of high school.

On weekdays, she left her house at 5:30 a.m. so she could be in the pool for 6:00 a.m. practice. Then came a full day of school, followed by after-school activities and homework, and finally, bedtime, usually between 11:30 p.m. and 12:30 a.m. Then she'd get up early the next morning and do it all over again.

"I really genuinely liked all the things I did, for the most part," Ruiz Chiu told me. At the same time, though, she felt the stress of preparing for college, and there were times it all seemed overwhelming. "I was very aware of college applications and making and building my resume," she recalled, "and making a good impression, and seeming like a very well-rounded student."

She tried not to think about the pressure she was feeling, but it continued to build. "I would go on runs and feel like, 'What if I just got hit by a car right now? Wouldn't that be nice?' I could sit in the hospital for a few weeks . . . At least I wouldn't have homework to do."

She didn't have the awareness or language to identify that she was depressed or recognize how severe it had gotten, she told me. Nor did her parents or her peers, many of whom had similar schedules.

"The kinds of conversations I would have with my friends would usually devolve into who's working harder, who's more tired—the comparison thing," she said. "I just remember feeling so stuck."

One evening in February 2002, about two-thirds of the way through her freshman year at Palo Alto High School, Ruiz Chiu reached the breaking point. Impulsively, she downed a bottle of Advil before joining her family for dinner. Her parents quickly realized something was wrong and rushed her to the hospital, leading to a mandatory seventy-two-hour psychiatric hold. "It was very traumatic," she said.

Her overdose was a turning point, Ruiz Chiu explained, although she acknowledged it wasn't a perfect 180-degree turn. After reevaluating her classes, she decided to switch from AP to regular-level science (her least favorite subject) but continued her other advanced-level classes. And while she ended up quitting the water polo team, she kept her other activities and added in track and field, which at least didn't have practice at dawn. "I think the difference was that I felt empowered to say no," she explained, "and to raise my hand when it was too much."

As she later characterized her experience, "My hard-driving, sleep-deprived daily routine exacerbated the pain and mood swings I was already experiencing as a hormonal teenager struggling to figure out who I was."[81]

★ ✦ ✱

In the two decades since Ruiz Chiu's attempted suicide, mental-health issues among adolescents, including depression, anxiety, suicidal ideation, and suicide attempts, have continued to rise. According to the CDC's national Youth Risk Behavior Survey, in 2005, 28.5 percent of high school students said they felt sad or hopeless. By 2019, the number had jumped to 36.7 percent. Even more worrisome, during the same timeframe, the percentage of high schoolers who said they'd seriously considered suicide rose from 16.9 to 18.8 percent, and those who'd actually attempted it increased from 8.4 to 8.9 percent.[82]

More recently, a public advisory by the US Surgeon General, which came out shortly before this book went to press, noted that the pandemic and other challenges have had a "devastating" effect on mental health for kids, teens, and young adults.

THE INTENSITY OF TEEN BRAINS (EVEN WITHOUT SLEEP LOSS)

While there are many contributing factors, both adolescence itself and sleep play important roles.

Before we get to the sleep piece or the pressures our teens are facing, let's take a peek under the hood at what's going on inside their brains.

First and foremost, their brains are still under development.

The extensive brain remodeling of the teen years is a massive project, as noted in Chapter 1, exceeded in scope only by what took place when they were babies.

Once it's complete, our teens will be able to make better decisions, focus their attention more effectively, and behave less impulsively, thanks to faster overall processing and the strengthened connections between neural cells and between brain regions. But all of this isn't fully completed until early adulthood.

Another critical point: this development takes place in different parts of the brain at different times.

The first part to rev up is what neuroscientist Jay Giedd has called "the hormone-fueled limbic system": the part of the brain responsible for emotions and reward seeking.[83] The result is a new intensity in how teens perceive the world: everything from a heightened responsiveness to dopamine (one of the key neurotransmitters for experiencing pleasure) to a greater tendency to act impulsively.

The braking system to help regulate all of this isn't yet in place, however, and won't be until the second phase of brain remodeling, during the middle teen years. As detailed by Temple University psychology professor Laurence Steinberg in *Age of Opportunity*, this phase is when the prefrontal cortex gets upgraded, which enhances "executive functioning"—everything from working memory, to being able to plan ahead, to the ability for abstract thought.[84]

Even after this, there's still one more phase of brain remodeling to strengthen connections *between* brain regions. It isn't until this connectivity is complete in early adulthood that teens possess reliable self-regulation, according to Steinberg. After this final upgrade, teens' "rational thought processes are less easily disrupted by fatigue, stress, or emotional arousal."

LACK OF SLEEP AND TEEN BRAINS

So, what happens when teens are functioning on too-little sleep? The intensity of what they're feeling is magnified.

That's true for all of us—not just teens.

"When we don't sleep well, our emotions run a little bit higher," UCLA neuroscientist Adriana Galván explained. "We're a little bit more reactive and impulsive."

The crucial difference is that teen brains are less equipped to cope with sleep loss. "As an adult, I have a mature prefrontal cortex that can help me regulate those emotions and keep them in check," Galván said. In teens, though, the prefrontal cortex is still under development, which means that "when their emotional reactivity brain region is in overdrive, they don't necessarily have the same additional neural tools to dampen that emotional response."

The Link between Sleep Loss and Anger and Other Intense Emotions

When teens don't get enough sleep, their emotions "run hotter"—including anger:

- As a 2020 study titled "Does Losing Sleep Unleash Anger?" found, the answer is yes: after getting less sleep than usual, US college students felt angrier the next day.[85]
- A study of more than 95,000 Japanese teenagers, published in 2016, showed those who hadn't gotten enough sleep were more likely to report feelings of intense anger.[86]
- In Sweden, a 2016 study of close to three thousand teens found those who slept less than seven hours were more likely to report feeling depressed, angry, or anxious.[87]

Inadequate sleep is also linked with depression. In a 2020 meta-analysis examining seventy-three previous studies conducted around the world, researchers found that not getting enough sleep increased teens' odds of feeling depressed by 62 percent.[88] Another study published that year focused on teens in the United Kingdom who had been diagnosed with depression. The teens not only went to bed later than their nondepressed counterparts, they also got less sleep overall, the researchers found.[89]

It's important to note that **the relationship between sleep and depression goes both ways**: sleeping poorly may contribute to depression, and depression may result in sleep disturbances.

SLEEP DEPRIVATION AND SUICIDE

As parents, we've long grown accustomed to being bombarded with information on how we can keep our kids safe in the world—everything from how and where they should sleep as newborns to how to protect them from being abducted. Perhaps the most gut-wrenching realization is that we can't always protect them from harm.

The highest risk of suicide our kids will ever face is during the timeframe from the preteen years to young adulthood. According to CDC data for 2019 and several years prior, suicide was the second-leading cause of death for preteens, teens, and young adults in the United States.[90]

As teens' sleep duration goes down, their suicide risk goes up. One study of middle and high schoolers in Fairfax County, Va., found that each hour of lost sleep was linked to a 42 percent increase in suicidal thoughts and a 58 percent increase in suicide attempts.[91]

Another study of close to 70,000 high school students found that teens who slept less than six hours were more than *three* times as likely to say they'd considered suicide, made a plan to attempt suicide, or actually attempted it compared to their counterparts who'd gotten at least eight hours of sleep.[92]

Finally, it's quite concerning, as noted earlier, that the percentage of high school students who have either contemplated or attempted suicide increased from 2005 to 2019, according to CDC data. That's even more unsettling juxtaposed against sleep findings from the CDC's 2019 national

Youth Risk Behavior Survey, which found that only 22.1 percent of US high school students said they got at least eight hours of sleep a night. That's a 9 percent drop from 2007.[93]

While mental-health experts are loath to oversimplify a complex problem, the relationship between sleep deprivation and suicidality is downright scary.

In teens' still-developing brains, "the threshold for making or acting on a decision is lower," Maida Chen, who directs the Sleep Center at Seattle Children's Hospital, explained. When sleep deprivation is layered in, the threshold drops even further.

"Looking back, I had been feeling suicidal for, probably, months," Ruiz Chiu told me when we spoke about her high school suicide attempt. "The whole winter leading up to the incident, I think I had been depressed, extremely fatigued, and exhausted. I do think sleep was a factor."

Even though all of those elements had been steadily building, it wasn't just Ruiz Chiu's sense of hopelessness and worsening depression that were heightened by sleep deprivation. What she characterizes as her "impulsive" decision to down a bottle of Advil was also likely influenced by her chronic lack of sleep.

In fact, **research shows that getting more sleep is one way to lower teens' suicide risk.** A meta-analysis of previous studies, published in 2018, highlighted what's called a dose-response relationship, showing that for every one-hour increase in adolescent sleep, the risk of planning suicide decreased 11 percent.[94]

BEING WELL RESTED BOOSTS POSITIVITY AND RESILIENCE

Of course, we don't need to wait for a crisis to know how much our teens' emotions are affected by sleep loss.

When we're well rested, worries seem less dire, tasks seem more doable, and people even seem less irritating. It's much easier to face the world and respond productively to both positive *and* negative input.

Someone who's sleep-deprived will interpret the identical stimuli differently than someone who's well rested. In *Why We Sleep*, neuroscientist Matthew Walker described an experiment in his lab in which participants were shown pictures of people's faces and asked to interpret their expressions along a continuum from friendly to threatening. Subjects who'd gotten a full night's sleep accurately identified the range of what was depicted. But when they were sleep-deprived, this ability fell away. "The sleep-deprived participants slipped into a default of fear bias, believing even gentle or somewhat friendly looking faces were menacing," Walker wrote.[95]

Even what we'd normally perceive as a positive experience often seems muted when we're running on fumes. This loss of pleasure, or more specifically, of the capacity to experience pleasure, has a clinical name: anhedonia. And it's a quality-of-life aspect for our teens, if they're trudging through their days, unable to find small moments of joy which might otherwise give them a boost.

Unfortunately, studies around the world have found this is far more likely when teens don't get enough sleep.

And when teens *do* get enough sleep? It's the opposite. Nancy Sin, an assistant professor of psychology at the University of British Columbia, has researched how sleep affects positive well-being. In one study, preteens and teens who said they slept better also rated their emotions as more positive (and said they had fewer arguments with their parents) than the kids who said they'd slept worse.[96]

Being well rested makes it easier to be attuned to positive experiences and serves as a catalyst, Sin told me. As she explained, "It's really about how much you can engage with your environment and take advantage of opportunities or create opportunities."

SLEEP AS AN EMOTIONAL BUFFER

Even when they're not in crisis, our teens are dealing with a multitude of daily stressors. As they navigate all of this—everything from friends (and frenemies) to homework deadlines, from minor irritations to major issues—their ability to cope is greater if they're well rested.

Getting enough sleep actually serves as an emotional buffer. In one intriguing study, published in 2020, ninth-graders used daily diaries for two weeks to track whether they'd experienced any ethnic or racial discrimination each day (and to what degree) and how they responded, along with their daily stress levels.[97]

After nights when students got more sleep and higher-quality sleep, they were better able to cope with discrimination and discrimination-related stress the following day. (Unfortunately, the relationship is bidirectional: discrimination also affects sleep, as we'll see in Chapter 9.)

Specifically, the teens who'd slept better reported using more active coping strategies, including problem solving and seeking out peer support. They also spent less time ruminating over what had occurred.

"Sleep can affect how we perceive stress and how we respond to it," said Tiffany Yip, chair of the psychology department at Fordham University and coauthor of the study.

It's not just sleeping well *before* a stressful day that matters; the amount of sleep teens get *after* also plays a key role in helping them rebound emotionally. In a study conducted in 2015, high schoolers in Maryland rated their daily mood and stress levels and their nightly sleep over a two-week period. When the teens got more sleep following a stressful day, they had less emotional "spillover" the next morning and rebounded more quickly. In fact, their positive feelings and emotions overall the next day were similar to what they reported following a low-stress day.[98]

To sum up, **when teens get enough sleep—and when that sleep is quality sleep—they feel better and are more emotionally resilient.** A 2020 study of more than a thousand teens and young adults in New Zealand and the United States found sleep quality and quantity were the two strongest predictors of depressive symptoms and of well-being.[99]

When it comes to sleep, "it's about replenishing," Marc Brackett, founder and director of the Yale Center for Emotional Intelligence, told me. "We need to replenish and if we don't, everything becomes more difficult."

WHEN SLEEP DEPRIVATION SEEMS NORMAL

With so many teens functioning in a haze of sleep deprivation, they're simply not as well equipped to handle the daily flood of emotions and stressors. Interpersonal slights are intensified. Challenges seem harder. And it's harder to discern the best path forward.

Unfortunately, far too many teens simply become accustomed to feeling this way.

"I felt really awful, but I just thought that was normal," Ruiz Chiu said.

Looking back, she wishes she'd been able to recognize all of this when she was still in school.

"I wish I could take my high school self and be like, 'Give me two weeks of your time . . . I'll clear your schedule so that you can get nine hours of sleep a night,'" Ruiz Chiu told me. "If I could have just shown myself what being rested actually could do for your quality of life and productivity, it probably would have made me more of a believer in sleep."

TEEN-SLEEP TAKEAWAYS

- Because their brains are still under development, teens' emotions are magnified.

- When teens are sleep-deprived, this is intensified: negative emotions such as anger run hotter, and positive emotions are muted.

- Suicide risk is highest during the timeframe including the teen years.

- Getting enough sleep is one way to boost mental health and help decrease suicidality.

- Sleep boosts emotional resilience and makes it easier to cope with stressors.

CHAPTER 5

Risky Behaviors and Unhealthy Habits

Let's take a quick quiz. Do the following seem like good ideas to you, or bad ones?

- Jumping off a roof
- Eating a cockroach
- Swimming with sharks

Abigail Baird, who's now a professor of psychological science at Vassar College, posed these and other scenarios to a group of adults and teens, using brain scans to illuminate how they arrived at their answers.[100]

You'll be relieved to know both teens and adults rated all three as bad ideas. But, the teens took longer to do so. Unlike the adults, for whom these activities elicited an immediate mental image and visceral response, the teens actually *thought* about the situations and then concluded they were dangerous. (As Baird and her coauthors noted, the teens' decision-making process relied on "less efficient brain networks.")

That's very much in keeping with the fact that teen brains are undergoing remodeling, as discussed in earlier chapters.

There's another key point about this experiment: it was conducted in a laboratory setting! In the real world, it's actually not that much of a leap to envision teens, in a group setting and perhaps fueled by alcohol or other substances, egging each other on to do only slightly less stupid things than jumping off a roof or eating a cockroach.

And, if the risky activity is actually a fun one—like flooring it to see how fast the car will go—they're more apt to have a visceral response that says, "Go for it!"

That's because teens are more apt to pursue what researchers term "reward- and sensation-seeking behaviors"—whether it's driving fast, experimenting with illegal substances, or accepting a dare.

In fact, their brains are uniquely configured to experience pleasure: the limbic system has revved up, as we saw in the previous chapter, and teen brains are flush with receptors for dopamine.

It isn't just that teens' mental braking systems haven't yet kicked in; the portion of the limbic system where the reward center is housed actually gets bigger during adolescence, then contracts as adulthood approaches, Temple University psychology professor Laurence Steinberg wrote in *Age of Opportunity*. Because of this, according to Steinberg, "Nothing . . . will ever feel as good as it did when you were a teenager."[101]

Wired for Excitement

Regardless of parenting and cultural expectations, teens all over the world seek out adventure and risk. When researchers looked at the behaviors of five thousand young people (ages ten to thirty) in eleven countries—China, Colombia, Cyprus, India, Italy, Jordan, Kenya, the Philippines, Sweden, Thailand, and the United States—they found that what they termed "sensation seeking" generally peaked in the mid to late teenage years. "Around the world," the authors concluded, "adolescence is a time when individuals are inclined to pursue exciting and novel experiences but have not yet fully developed the capacity to keep impulsive behavior in check."[102]

WHAT ABOUT WHEN TEENS ARE SLEEP-DEPRIVED?

With teen brains already wired for risk, sleep deprivation adds yet another layer of intensity.

It isn't just that sleep-starved teens are more affected by positive cues and potential rewards, though. They also make riskier choices.

The effects of too-little sleep don't take long to kick in: one in-lab study showed that after just one night of very restricted sleep (four hours), teenagers demonstrated poorer inhibitory control (the ability to control impulsive responses) and "greater risk-taking behavior."[103]

As noted in Chapter 4, we *all* function worse when we're sleep-deprived. (As UCLA neuroscientist Adriana Galván has written, "The brain processes identical emotional, rewarding, or cognitive information differently when it has been deprived of sleep.")[104] Compared to adults, however, the effect on teens' behavior can be even more pronounced.

A LINK BETWEEN SLEEP AND CRIME

Ryan Meldrum, an associate professor and criminologist at Florida International University, has researched the role sleep loss plays in adolescent crime.

"[It's] kind of a sequential process or cascading effect," he told me, given that lack of sleep impedes teens' judgment and self-control. That's a key point, Meldrum explained: "Self-control is one of, if not *the*, strongest predictor of engagement in delinquency and crime."

In one study, published in 2015, Meldrum and his coauthors found sleep deprivation was linked to low self-control, which in turn was linked to delinquency—everything from vandalism to attacking someone with a weapon.[105]

There's another way poor sleep contributes to risky behaviors, he found: it can make teens more receptive to peer influences.[106] (On the flip side, he noted that **getting enough sleep can be a protective factor against susceptibility to peer influence**.)

Intriguingly, later school start times may be a way to address this, and not just because they enable teens to get more sleep. When schools start later, they generally let out later. This may help reduce the amount of time teens spend in the afternoons engaged in "unstructured socializing with peers," Meldrum said, which plays a role in delinquency.[107] There's typically an increase in youth crime at about 3:00 or 4:00 p.m., and the theory is that later school release times cut into this window of opportunity, he noted.

Data published by the Office of Juvenile Justice and Delinquency Prevention (part of the US Department of Justice) underscores that there is indeed a link between the timing of when school lets out and when crimes occur. On school days, violent crimes by under-eighteen-year-olds peak at 3:00 p.m.—far higher than any other time of day, including weekends. "Violent crimes by juveniles occur most frequently in the hours immediately following the close of school on school days," the analysts wrote.[108]

Lastly, how sleep-deprived teens are—another area Meldrum has studied—also affects risky behaviors. He and a coauthor analyzed data from the 2011 national Youth Risk Behavior Survey, which included responses from more than 15,000 high schoolers. Overall, one-sixth of the respondents reported carrying a weapon (defined as a gun, knife, or club) at least once in the past thirty days. Of these, the teens who averaged less than five hours of sleep on school nights were 172 percent more likely to have done so than teens who reported getting at least eight hours of sleep.[109]

SUBSTANCE USE

Compared to adults, **adolescents are more prone to addiction**, and not just because they're more likely to take risks and seek out pleasure. They're also quicker to learn new skills and behaviors, thanks to the teen brain refinement taking place: the more often specific neurons are used, the stronger the connections between them become.

Regardless of what the behavior is, "Every time you do it, you're reinforcing [it]," Galván told me. "You're strengthening that synapse, and you may be recruiting new synapses and creating new synapses to support that behavior."

"Moreover, compared to adults, teens who do become addicted may have a harder time overcoming that addiction," she said.

As with other risky teen behaviors, substance use has been linked to lack of sleep. One study of more than 2,500 teens in California, published in 2015, revealed that teens who reported later bedtimes and less total nightly sleep in the past month were far more likely to have consumed alcohol or used marijuana during the same timeframe.[110]

Another study, published in 2018, looked at a variety of risky behaviors. After analyzing the responses from more than 67,000 high schoolers, the authors concluded that those who reported getting less sleep on school nights were correspondingly more likely to report alcohol, marijuana, or other drug use in the past thirty days.[111]

With adolescents already more prone to addiction, the heightened risk from sleep deprivation is enough to send shivers down any parent's spine. (There is a bright side, though: the teens who said they got at least eight hours of nightly sleep had the lowest odds for substance use.[112])

STIMULANTS, CAFFEINE, AND ENERGY DRINKS

There's a similar dynamic at play when it comes to stimulant use, including prescription medications such as Ritalin or Adderall. While teens may turn to them as a way to stay up late and sharpen their focus, these medications are "capable of trapping adolescents in a cycle of habitual use and addiction," neuroscientist Frances Jensen wrote in *The Teenage Brain*.[113]

The most common, as you'd expect, is **caffeine, which is consumed by about 80 percent of teens.**[114]

"Caffeine is one of the best stimulants we have," Wendy Troxel, a senior behavioral and social scientist at the RAND Corporation, told me. Even so, she calls it a "compensatory strategy" better suited to workers whose jobs prevent them from getting enough sleep than it is for teens.

"It's used as a performance enhancer and to compensate for sleep loss in populations where we know sleep deprivation is sort of a job requirement," Troxel said, "whether it be a physician working in the ER or a night-shift worker or a soldier . . . but that's not really where we should be going with otherwise healthy teenagers."

Caffeine helps counteract sleepiness by temporarily blocking the brains receptors for adenosine, which prompts feeling sleepy. However, because caffeine can overstimulate those same receptors, taking in too much can backfire and make you feel anxious or jittery, Harris Lieberman, a research psychologist with the US Army Research Institute of Environmental Medicine, explained.

"As you get a higher and higher dose, you go from a desirable behavioral effect of increased alertness to what essentially is an overstimulated status," said Lieberman, who's conducted extensive research on caffeine.

Another potential pitfall: consuming too much caffeine or doing so later in the day can make it hard to fall asleep at night.

It's easy to see how this can become a vicious cycle: caffeine use delays sleep, leading to too few hours of sleep, which then results in sleepiness the following day and, likely, more caffeine.

Not surprisingly, a study published in 2018 found that teens' top reason for consuming energy drinks was to compensate for lack of sleep.[115]

It's worrisome when caffeine becomes an ongoing coping strategy, Lieberman pointed out. "Caffeine should never be considered as a substitute for sleep. It's a tool if you can't get enough sleep."

So, what's a good guideline for teens? About 100 milligrams of caffeine per day, he said. That's the amount in an eight-ounce cup of coffee, and, perhaps more relevant for teens, the general amount in a small energy drink.

However, many energy drinks, especially larger ones, may contain far more than that. Unlike soft drinks, which are classified as beverages and therefore regulated by the US Food and Drug Administration, most energy drinks are classified as dietary supplements. That's a key difference because it means **energy drinks, unlike soft drinks, don't have a maximum level of caffeine they're allowed to contain** (as measured by volume or by serving).

There's an additional concern about energy drinks, which is that they're frequently consumed with alcohol. In a study of US college students, one in ten reported having had at least one energy drink mixed with alcohol in the past two weeks,[116] a potent combination that can result in feeling "wide-awake drunk."

When it comes to stimulants to help teens cope with sleep loss, "It's a slippery slope," Troxel said. "There's something to keep you awake, and there's something to help you sleep. And that's a slippery slope at a time in development when we know there's skyrocketing risk for the onset of substance-use problems."

Underlying all of this is the mindset of coping with sleep deprivation rather than addressing it, she added. "Instead of treating the problem, 'just take something for it' [is] a dangerous proposition, and a dangerous sort of belief system to be teaching our kids."

SLEEP AND EATING HABITS

There's another aspect of caffeinated beverages that's often overlooked: energy drinks, sodas, and frothy coffee drinks are usually loaded with sugar and calories. (A Starbucks venti caramel Frappuccino, for example, has 470 calories and 72 grams of sugar.)

These drinks likely play a role in contributing to obesity risks for sleep-deprived teens. Troxel noted that there's an "indirect path, potentially through increasing sugar consumption, that goes along with the caffeine." There's also a directional association, she pointed out: "Insufficient sleep can lead to increased risk for obesity, particularly in children and adolescents."

Studies have shown when we're sleep-deprived, we feel hungrier,[117] and we're also more drawn to sugary, higher-fat foods.[118] That's true for everyone, not just teens. In one experiment conducted in Japan, young adults who'd gotten just five hours of sleep for three nights in a row showed a preference for sweeter foods—the equivalent, the researchers noted, of opting to add an additional 1½ tablespoons of sugar to a cup of coffee.[119] Similar results were found in a study of US teens who were restricted to six and a half hours in bed for five nights in a row. Not only did the teens rate sweets and desserts as more appealing, the number of servings they consumed increased by more than 50 percent.[120]

Finally, researchers have found that teens who don't get enough sleep are more likely to be overweight. One study funded by the National Institutes of Health showed that the teens who reported getting the least amount of sleep (under six hours on school nights) were also more likely to be obese.[121]

Lack of sleep is just one driver of obesity, but it's an important one, researchers note. (Neuroscientist Matthew Walker has put it in stronger terms, writing, "The epidemic of insufficient sleep is very likely a key contributor to the epidemic of obesity."[122]) Against the backdrop of the latest numbers—according to the CDC's 2019 national Youth Risk Behavior Survey, close to a third of high school students are considered overweight or obese—the role of sleep deprivation shouldn't be overlooked.

IMMUNITY AND HEALING

What about immunity and other aspects of physical well-being? Again, it turns out that sleep is involved. Without adequate sleep, wounds heal more slowly,[123] and there's even a likely link between sleep and the body's defenses against illness.

In a memorable study, researchers squeezed nasal drops containing rhinovirus (the virus for the common cold) up the noses of sleep-deprived adults. Those adults were more likely to come down with a cold than their non-sleep-deprived counterparts. (Specifically, participants who'd gotten less than five hours of nightly sleep the prior week had a 45 percent chance of developing a cold after being exposed to the virus. For those who'd gotten at least seven hours of sleep each night, the risk was only 17 percent.)

"Short sleep was more important than any other factor in predicting subjects' likelihood of catching cold," the study's lead author, sleep researcher Aric Prather, said when the findings were released in 2015.[124]

Sleep and Vaccines

Getting enough sleep may be a key way to bolster vaccine effectiveness. In a 2021 study focusing on flu vaccines, Prather, an associate professor of psychiatry and behavioral sciences at the University of California, San Francisco (UCSF), had a group of healthy college freshmen keep sleep diaries both before and after receiving a standard flu vaccine. The results showed that getting less sleep the two nights prior to getting vaccinated was associated with lower antibody responses both one month and four months afterwards (specifically for one of the main flu strains they were being vaccinated against). As noted in the study's conclusion, the results "suggest that sleep may play an important role in preparing the immune system . . . to mount an effective response."[125]

Also of note: Prather was a principal investigator for a recently completed study examining how sleep and other variables affect long-term responses to COVID-19 vaccines. (The results of that study are forthcoming as of this writing.)[126]

All of this notwithstanding, there's also the low-grade, persistent sense of not feeling well many sleep-deprived teens face, and it's one that unfortunately ends up getting normalized.

"I just always had . . . a chronic state of [being] about to get a cold," Taylor Ruiz Chiu, the former Palo Alto High School student, said. "My body got kind of used to feeling bad."

Normalizing feeling bad isn't what we want for our teens—nor are any of the other behaviors covered in this chapter. Their brains may be wired to seek rewards and take risks, but we can help keep our teens from amping this up any further, as well as boost their resistance and help them feel healthier.

And it all starts with a good night's sleep.

TEEN-SLEEP TAKEAWAYS

- Teen brains are already primed for risk-taking and pleasure-seeking behaviors, and being sleep-deprived intensifies this.

- The pathway for addiction is stronger during the teen years.

- Drinking caffeine (including in energy drinks) can create a vicious cycle.

- Lack of sleep boosts appetite, especially for sugary foods.

- Being well rested promotes immunity and healing.

CHAPTER 6

Sleepwalking through School

Hearing about early start times is one thing; living them is another. In 2007, then-junior Sage Snider and three friends decided to capture the experience with a "day in the life" documentary for their media-studies class.

The film is poignant. There's a shot of buses trundling along in the dark, followed by footage of students trudging into the high school main building, its brightly lit interior a sharp contrast to the still-black sky. "We have buses in this county picking up students before 6:00 a.m. in order to get them to their high schools," the principal acknowledges in the film.

The camera then peeks inside several first-period (7:17 a.m.) classes, showing countless students slumped over their desks, fast asleep. In one class, the AP US history teacher tries in vain to keep the class awake— several students startle as he yells suddenly, only to settle right back down again.

That wasn't an unusual occurrence, Sage said; as a student in his class, there were many days when she herself fell asleep.

Students elsewhere in the country remember similar struggles to stay awake.

In Pennsylvania, after racing out of the house to catch the 7:00 a.m. bus to Radnor High School, Annabel Zhao often used her backpack as a makeshift pillow so she could nap on the way to school.

And in California, "I was just not grasping concepts as easily as I would have been when rested," Taylor Ruiz Chiu told me, recalling her high school days in Palo Alto. "That made me feel like I was stupider, and maybe I didn't deserve to be in these honors classes."

It's now been more than forty-five years since the Stanford Summer Sleep Camp was founded. In that time, there's been a mountain of supporting evidence for later school start times, documenting the implications not just for academic performance but for other school-related behaviors as well.

Teens may be tardy or absent. They may be asleep in class. Or they may be going through the motions, but, as pioneering sleep researcher Mary Carskadon has written, "Their brains are at home on their pillows."[127]

WHAT IT'S LIKE FOR TEACHERS

Teaching a roomful of semi-comatose students is far from ideal. "I definitely worked harder during first hour to engage students," retired health teacher Pacy Erck said, recalling the years prior to Edina High School's start-time change. "As a teacher, you engage back and forth—it's a two-way street. They weren't saying anything unless I initiated it."

In fact, Erck said, "There were some students who were quite resentful of my outgoing perkiness at 7:30 in the morning."

After Edina shifted its start time, "The biggest change for me literally was that first period," Erck told me. "The students were just so much more engaged in a positive way."

Seattle biology teacher Cindy Jatul noticed a similar transformation at Roosevelt High School after the district's 2016 shift to an 8:45 a.m. start time. "You just feel it when you come into the school in the morning," she said. "It feels like a more upbeat atmosphere."

Feedback from students and their families was also positive, said Jatul, a former nurse practitioner who started advocating for later start times when her daughter entered adolescence. "There were students who really thanked me personally because of the improvement in their mental health."

At the first back-to-school night after the shift, Jatul invited parents to share written comments. "The majority were like, 'This is great—this means my kids are human again [and] we can relate.'"

The reason, as documented in a study involving Jatul's students: teens were getting more sleep!

Both before and after the start-time change, researchers documented students' reported and actual sleep. Data was gathered the spring semester prior to the shift and again a year later. In both cases, sophomores in biology classes at Roosevelt and at a second Seattle high school, Franklin, completed sleep diaries and questionnaires. Subsets of the students wore actigraphy watches for a two-week period to record their sleep. "It was a new cohort of kids, but they were taking the exact same classes in the exact same schools," University of Washington biology professor Horacio de la Iglesia, one of the study's coauthors, pointed out.

Those results, published in 2018, showed students slept an additional thirty-four minutes each school night.[128]

Narrowing the Education Equity Gap

The later start was particularly beneficial at Seattle's Franklin High School, where 68 percent of students were non-White and 88 percent came from economically disadvantaged households.

At Franklin, attendance went up and tardiness went down—changes de la Iglesia characterized as a "leveling effect." With the 7:50 a.m. start time, both absences and tardies had been higher at Franklin than at Roosevelt. But with the 8:45 a.m. start time, those gaps narrowed significantly.

The Seattle findings added to a growing body of research showing **later school start times have equity implications.**

In one influential study, Finley Edwards, then a visiting assistant professor of economics at Colby College, evaluated middle school start times and student achievement in Wake County, North Carolina. The schools' start times ranged from 7:30 a.m. to 8:15 a.m. (with a few outliers starting as late as 8:45 a.m.). He found later start times resulted in higher standardized test scores, especially in math, with economically disadvantaged students showing the most improvement.[129]

As sleep researchers Lauren Hale and Wendy Troxel have written, "Healthy school start times are not only a critical public health issue, but also an important social justice issue."[130]

That's because teens of color and teens who live in lower-income households or neighborhoods tend to sleep worse than their counterparts (as we'll cover in Chapter 9) and may face additional hurdles. When they're also faced with too-early start times, which further erode their sleep, these disadvantages are further compounded. **However, starting schools later in the morning is a proven, effective way to help address these disparities.**

ATTENDANCE AND TARDIES

The link between later starts and reduced absences and tardies seen at Seattle's Franklin High School has been well documented around the country, dating all the way back to some of the first schools to change their start times based on the research in the late 1990s.

In Minneapolis, where start times were delayed from 7:15 a.m. to 8:40 a.m. in 1997, the University of Minnesota's Kyla Wahlstrom conducted the first longitudinal study to measure the impact. Among her findings: for students who attended more than one high school over the course of their schooling (a disruption often due to personal circumstances, and a stressful change layered on top of all the "standard" high school stressors), **later starts boosted attendance.**[131]

In Glens Falls, New York, **unexcused tardies dropped 20 percent** after the local high school moved its start time from 7:45 a.m. to 8:30 a.m.[132]

And at twenty-nine high schools in seven states that moved their start times to 8:30 a.m. or later, researchers found **average attendance rates increased from 90 percent to 94 percent.**[133]

SLEEPY KIDS AND TRUANCY

When students don't show up for class, things can quickly spiral downward given the toll chronic absenteeism takes on learning.

Moreover, even if sleep deprivation is what's causing those absences, well-intentioned truancy laws aren't necessarily the right approach.

In the state of Washington, for instance, schools are required to file truancy petitions for juvenile court if students have seven unexcused absences in a month or ten in an academic year.

Maida Chen of Seattle Children's Hospital told me that many of her patients at the sleep center were kids who'd been categorized as truant. They'd get caught in an endless process, she told me, with required truancy classes, along with trips to see her in order to get a medical excuse for the absences, taking up even *more* time and causing even *more* stress for families. "We had, like, a zero percent success rate in converting these kids," she said.

On one of her first visits to the Seattle Public Schools administration building to advocate for later start times, she recalled passing a room where a truancy class was in progress and spotting two of her patients there.

In fact, it was often the truancy officers who flagged the issue, she said: "They would recognize that the kids were so sleepy during the day, that this was contributing to the problem."

IT'S HARD TO LEARN IF YOU'RE ZONED OUT

It's no surprise that **when teens get more sleep, they're more awake and ready to learn.**

"For jumping right into *Beowulf* or *Macbeth*," high school teacher Mona Madron explained in Sage Snider's student film, "you know, you really have to have a level of consciousness before you can understand that literature."

Being able to engage with the information and stay focused—what researchers term "sustained attention"—is far less likely when teens can barely stay awake.

It's also difficult for sleepy teens to remember what they've learned, neurologist Chris Winter, author of *The Sleep Solution,* told me. "REM sleep is very important for memory consolidation. It really helps in that transition to more stable memory," he said, "versus something that's being held transiently and is going to be flushed away pretty quickly."

How Sleep Affects Learning

Being sleep-deprived affects learning in three key ways, according to Carskadon:[134]

- It hampers the process of *acquiring* new information (when students are learning in class, or reading or studying on their own).
- It lessens the likelihood of *retaining* the information (which occurs during sleep, when newly acquired information is consolidated, stabilized, and strengthened).
- It impairs the ability to *retrieve* the information (when students are trying to recall what they've learned so they can build on concepts, complete homework, or take tests).

WHAT ABOUT GRADES?

In an extensive study looking at sleep and academic performance, the University of Minnesota's Kyla Wahlstrom examined data from more than nine thousand students at eight schools in Colorado, Minnesota, and Wyoming.[135]

In five of the six districts studied, she found statistically significant increases in students' GPAs in core courses after the schools shifted to later start times.

As she concluded, **"The evidence shows that the later the start time, the greater the academic benefits."**[136]

Being able to document this was a turning point, she said, because it helped provide superintendents who were following the issue with some of the evidence they needed. "I get lots of calls from superintendents," she told me. Prior to that study, "they did not care, oftentimes, that these other outcomes were so positive if there wasn't also an academic benefit, because they could not sell it to the school board without an academic reason for making the change."

More recently, the Seattle study by the University of Washington's de la Iglesia found that grades rose by 4.5 percent after the start-time change.

That's a "huge increment," he said, given that it was in "the very same classes, [with] the very same teachers."

ADHD and Sleep Deprivation

In the twenty-year period from 1997 to 2016, the number of children and teens in the United States diagnosed with attention deficit hyperactivity disorder (ADHD) increased dramatically, to about 10 percent of all four- to seventeen-year-olds.[137]

For kids with ADHD, difficulty paying attention and staying on task can make it hard to stay focused on schoolwork. Argelinda Baroni, who codirects the Child and Adolescent Sleep Program at Hassenfeld Children's Hospital at NYU Langone, has written that this inattention includes "[careless] mistakes, difficulty sustaining attention and following instructions, distractibility, and frequent daydreaming."[138]

Looking again at this list, you may also notice that **some of these symptoms are the same ones caused by sleep deprivation!** In a study published in 2012, teachers in Canada were asked to use an ADHD screening tool to rate various behaviors of a group of elementary school students. None of the kids actually had ADHD, but some had gotten more sleep than their peers. It turned out that the kids who'd slept the least were the most likely to exhibit ADHD-related symptoms, including cognitive problems and inattentiveness.[139]

What's more, ADHD is often associated with sleep issues. "Between 50 percent and 70 percent of kids with ADHD have some form of sleep disorder," Baroni told me, which in turn can exacerbate symptoms.

In fact, sleep problems can "precede, predict, and significantly contribute to" ADHD symptoms, as clinical psychologist Reut Gruber—who directs the Attention Behavior and Sleep Lab at the Douglas Mental Health University Institute in Montreal—and her colleagues wrote in a 2021 research review.[140]

Finally, the medications used to treat ADHD, which are generally stimulants, can also cause sleep issues, Baroni said.

The bottom line? Sleep deprivation and ADHD are often intertwined. They contribute to and amplify one another. If your teen has ADHD, it's even more important to pay attention to sleep. And, if your teen has ADHD-like symptoms, you may want to evaluate whether sleep issues are playing a role.

GRADUATION AND BEYOND

Along with boosting attendance and grades, later start times increase graduation rates—a key predictor of future success.

Kids who aren't absent or tardy aren't missing as much in-class instruction, and kids who aren't struggling to stay awake are absorbing more of what they're learning.

In the same study looking at the effect of later start times on attendance at twenty-nine high schools, the researchers also examined graduation rates. (All of the high schools had shifted their start times to 8:30 a.m. or later.) Before the shift, the average graduate rate was 79 percent; two years later, it had surged to 88 percent.[141]

WHAT ABOUT THE FINANCIAL IMPACT?

Even if viewed narrowly as just a financial decision, later school start times make sense. In 2015, Teny Shapiro, then an assistant professor of economics at Santa Clara University, analyzed the costs and benefits of later start times. She found the improvements resulting from a one-hour start-time delay were equivalent to those from reducing class size by one-third.[142]

Another important consideration: In some states, school funding is tied to attendance. Given the research showing that later start times translate into higher attendance, **this means more money for schools.**

There are longer-term gains too, with increased graduation rates and other benefits fueling economic growth. An influential 2017 RAND Corporation report coauthored by Wendy Troxel estimated that **shifting start times to 8:30 a.m. could boost the US economy by $83 billion within ten years**. The projected gains were based on the subsequent economic impact of increased academic performance and graduation rates on future earnings, as well as the related future economic benefits resulting from fewer car crashes.[143] These gains would greatly outweigh likely short-term costs associated with changing start times, such as those for transportation (covered in more detail in Chapter 14).

And of course, it's not all about test scores, or money. Teens may still be getting good grades and appear successful even when they're sleep-deprived, but it can come at a personal cost, as we've seen in earlier chapters.

In California, when researchers studied a group of high schoolers to determine the optimal amount of sleep for academic achievement and for mental health, the results were quite telling. The students needed seven to seven and a half hours of sleep a night to achieve the highest levels of academic performance. **But it was the teens who got more than an additional hour of sleep—eight and three-quarters to nine hours per night—who had the lowest levels of mental-health issues such as moodiness, feeling of worthlessness, anxiety, and depression.** (Note: while all of the teens in the study were Mexican American, the authors note that the achievement results mirrored those from other broader studies. Regardless, these results are a sobering reminder of the mental-health implications of sleep.)[144]

LATER STARTS ARE OVERDUE

Given everything now known about teen sleep—along with the abundance of evidence showing that later start times *work*—it's clear teens shouldn't be starting school at the crack of dawn.

And when schools don't make the change—for myriad reasons, often logistical (as we'll cover in Chapter 14), it's the teens who bear the consequences. Back in 1999, the *New York Times* captured the tearful reaction of fifteen-year-old Elizabeth, in Westchester County, New York, who'd just found out later start times had been voted down and she'd have to keep getting to school by 7:15 a.m.[145]

"Why is it," she asked her mother, "that people around here don't like kids?"

TEEN-SLEEP TAKEAWAYS

- Teens don't learn as well when they're sleep-deprived.

- When schools shift to later start times, teens get more sleep.

- Other benefits from later start times: higher grades and graduation rates, and fewer absences and tardies.

- Later start times help narrow education equity gaps and are also economically beneficial.

- Sleep deprivation and ADHD are often intertwined.

CHAPTER 7

Sleep and Sports

For a decade after joining the NBA, Andre Iguodala followed the sleep schedule he'd established as an undergraduate at the University of Arizona. At night, he'd stay awake until 3:00 or 4:00 a.m. playing video games. In the morning, he'd get up and head to practice. And in the afternoon, he'd try to squeeze in a long nap.

"It was around my tenth or eleventh year in the NBA [when] I said, 'Hey, I gotta tackle this issue,' " he recounted in a TIME 100 Health Summit talk in 2020.

Iguodala, who'd joined the Golden State Warriors in 2013, turned to Cheri Mah, a physician scientist at the Human Performance Center at the University of California, San Francisco, to help him overhaul his sleep habits.

"We took a holistic approach at looking at Andre's sleep," Mah said during the 2020 talk. That included reevaluating not just the timing of his sleep but the duration (which was often less than six hours), along with his routine—everything from his sleeping environment to his caffeine intake.

The results, even for an already phenomenal athlete, were stunning: His three-point performance more than doubled, his points per minute increased by 29 percent, and his free-throw percentage went up by 9 percent.

"When I first saw [the results], I was like, 'Whoa,' " he said.

And there were other changes too: "I could actually remember the games where I got a good night's rest more so than I could the ones [when] it wasn't really an optimal night of sleep," he said.

SLEEP AS A COMPETITIVE ADVANTAGE

Iguodala may be one of her most visible clients, but over the last decade or so, Mah has worked with athletes and teams from the NBA, the NFL, the NHL, and Major League Baseball. She's also seen the focus on sleep as a way to enhance performance become far more common.

"There's been a change in mindset that has been really fascinating to watch over the last ten years," she told me.

Mah's 2011 study of Stanford basketball players—and the dramatic improvements they posted after improving their sleep—helped jump-start the change.[146]

As part of the study, the players aimed to spend at least ten hours a night in bed, with a goal of improving the amount they slept each night from their baseline average (which was less than seven hours). Not only did their sleep increase to close to eight and a half hours per night, they posted impressive gains on the court: a 9 percent increase in successful free throws and three-point field goals, as well as faster sprint times.

When they're sleep-deprived, even "phenomenal" athletes like Iguodala "just aren't at their peak performance level," Mah said.

Neurologist Chris Winter, author of *The Rested Child*, shares a similar message with the professional and high school athletes he advises, frequently drawing on Mah's results to illustrate the potential impact optimal sleep can have.

"With a lot of pro teams I work with, I'll look at their last twenty games, and their win-loss record," he told me. "We look at it as it was, and we look at it with 9 percent more three pointers and free throws made. It's unbelievable how many more wins it puts in your column."

In another telling study, researchers analyzed the timing of tweets by NBA players, focusing on those who were sending tweets after 11:00 p.m. the night before a game. Players who were up late (as evidenced by their time-stamped tweets) generally performed worse compared to their stats for other games, the researchers found, including making fewer of their shots.[147]

Winter's own study of Major League Baseball players found sleepiness was strongly correlated with longevity in the league: three years down the road, the players who had initially reported the highest levels of sleepiness were the least likely to still be playing.[148]

"We were shocked by how linear the relationship was," he said when the results were released in 2013.

"That's a theme I've seen over the years," Winter told me, adding that athletes who make sleep a priority "just enjoy longer and more sustainable success."

Both Mah and Winter see sleep as foundational for high school athletes as well.

As Winter puts it, "I can promise you if you start now as a ninth-grader or tenth-grader and you really make sleep a priority, you will be a different athlete a year or two years from now."

Maintaining Eligibility

Academic standards for eligibility vary by state, but generally require athletes to meet a minimum grade threshold. In California and Florida, for instance, the minimum required GPA is a 2.0; in Texas, students must be passing all classes with a grade of 70 or higher. Particularly for academically at-risk athletes, getting enough sleep can help improve grades (as seen in the previous chapter).

SLEEPY ATHLETES ARE MORE LIKELY TO GET INJURED

The reality, of course, is most high school athletes *aren't* getting optimal sleep, as much as they might want to. "It's often overlooked and sacrificed, just given the busy schedules," Mah said.

Lack of sleep, which affects everything from coordination to response time, is "a risk factor for injury," Bianca Edison, an attending physician in the Children's Orthopaedic Center at Children's Hospital Los Angeles (CHLA), said.

She pointed to a 2014 study, by a team including CHLA researchers, which tracked sleep and sports activities of secondary school athletes at a Los Angeles private school. Of the students who slept less than eight hours (the minimum recommended amount), 65 percent sustained injuries, compared to just 31 percent of their better-rested classmates.[149]

Once athletes are injured, there are ramifications: everything from lost playing time to medical costs to increased risks for subsequent injuries.

During the 2018–19 school year, the estimated number of high school sports injuries topped 1.3 million. (This estimate, from the National High

School Sports-Related Injury Surveillance System, is calculated based on injuries reported by a nationally representative sample of high schools.) The injuries ranged from strains and sprains to concussions to wrist fractures; more than a third resulted in lost playing time ranging from one to three weeks, and nearly one-fourth kept athletes out even longer.

About Concussions

Nearly 20 percent of the high school sports injuries reported to the National High School Sports-Related Injury Surveillance System for 2018–19 were concussions. That equates to **more than 245,000 estimated concussions!**

Which Sports Have the Most Concussions?

They're not all happening in football, although it does top the list (based on the reported data for the 2013–14 through 2017–18 school years). Of the sports with the highest concussion rates, three of the top seven were girls' sports:[150]

- Boys' tackle football
- Girls' soccer
- Boys' ice hockey
- Boys' lacrosse
- Girls' basketball
- Boys' wrestling
- Girls' lacrosse

That said, participants in all of the twenty sports studied—everything from track and field to cheerleading to swimming—sustained concussions, the authors reported.

With sleep and sports-related concussions, there's a bidirectional relationship, Michael Grandner, director of the Sleep and Health Research Program at the University of Arizona, has written.[151]

First, poor sleep increases concussion risk. As Grandner and his coauthors found in a 2019 study, NCAA Division I athletes who reported having excessive daytime sleepiness and/or clinically moderate-to-severe insomnia at least twice during the past month had a higher risk of sustaining a sports-related concussion.[152]

Second, concussions themselves can trigger poor sleep. "A lot of things are thrown off, which filters down into your sleep being thrown off," Grandner told me. "There are lots of pathways from concussion to sleep problems," he said, which include daytime sleepiness and insomnia.

The final and most serious reason why concussed teens shouldn't rush back to play: the potentially catastrophic consequences of sustaining another concussion before the symptoms of the first one have subsided. (That's why every state has passed concussion return-to-play laws, spurred by the Zackery Lystedt Law in Washington, named for a teen who ended up permanently disabled after this exact scenario.)

THE SLEEP-RECOVERY CONNECTION

From a healing and recovery standpoint, sleep—which is when growth hormone, essential for recovery and growth, is secreted—plays an essential role.

Also important: the immune system activities that occur while we slumber. "The immune system is operating in the background all the time, when we talk about regeneration, and repair and recovery, and the lifecycle of the cell," Grandner said. It's not sleep itself "that builds the muscles back, or clears the waste," he explained, but that "sleep is the context" for this maintenance.

If you're not getting proper sleep, he added, "the system doesn't work as it's intended to."

Recovery from Injuries

Getting injured can also put "a real strain on your anxiety levels," particularly for kids who see being an athlete as part of their identity, Edison of CHLA told me.

Even though those kids may be itching to get back out there, she urged them to take enough time to recover and to get enough sleep.

Shoot for "the latter end of the spectrum," she said. So, for older teens like high schoolers, who tend to fall at the lower half of the eight-to-ten-hour recommended range, "Aim for nine [hours] instead of eight."

When teens don't get enough sleep, they aren't providing adequate time for their muscles to store glycogen, which is their quick energy source, Edison explained. "Fatigue levels correlate with glycogen depletion, which affects their ability to perform at their peak level or at a high intensity," Edison said.

Building up those glycogen stores is even more important when teens are recovering from an injury, she pointed out. "With the proper levels in place, when you're ready to go, you can do all those high-powered moves and you're not exhausting your body to possibly sustain another injury. Because if your muscles aren't at that peak level of strength and stability," Edison said, "you can end up with another injury."

Recovery from Workouts

The pressure from coaches—and from peers—can be powerful, but building in enough downtime for rest and recovery is also important.

Your body uses rest not just to rebuild but to "rebuild back better," Grandner explained.

This may mean trying to plan ahead, sleep-wise, to recover after intense workouts.

If, for example, you're doing a hard lifting session or plyometric workout, you're creating micro-tears in the muscle, Edison explained, adding that getting proper rest afterwards is what helps your body "rebuild and strengthen." When athletes don't get enough recovery sleep, "those small micro-tears can remain torn, which then increases your risk to tear them even more," she said.

As part of a focus on helping teens get more sleep, some schools are even taking steps to curb nighttime sports practices and games: At Biddeford High School in Maine, before-school and late-night practices were both banned in 2016.

Even so, the reality for many teen athletes is a schedule that often includes nighttime practices or games. Having a wind-down routine can help, but it may also be time to reevaluate your teen's overall commitments. Are they doing club sports in addition to school-sponsored leagues? Do they jump right from one sport season to another (often overlapping) one?

The takeaway advice from UCSF physician scientist Cheri Mah for high school athletes is to develop their approach to sleep and really be intentional about it. "The earlier they can establish this strategy . . . I think that will be the biggest advantage to them long term."

SLEEP STRATEGIES FOR TEEN ATHLETES

All of this may sound daunting, but even incremental sleep improvements make a difference. "Small things will add up over time," said Mah.

She described the "three buckets" of sleep to concentrate on:

1. Duration: even if it's just half an hour more than what you were getting the previous week, it counts!
2. Quality: find one action you can take, whether it's shifting technology use so it's earlier in the evening or starting a wind-down routine. (For more on this, see Chapter 11.)
3. Timing and schedule: if your bedtime typically varies by several hours, try to narrow that window so you're going to sleep at a more consistent time.

TEEN-SLEEP TAKEAWAYS

- Sleep boosts athletic performance.

- Even small improvements to sleep can make a difference.

- Because it's linked to academic performance, getting enough sleep can help athletes maintain their eligibility to play.

- The likelihood of injury is higher for sleep-deprived athletes.

- Sleep plays an essential role in recovery after injuries and after hard workouts and practices.

- After a concussion, allow enough time for recovery (including sleep). Skimping on this leaves teens vulnerable to long-term consequences, including subsequent concussions.

CHAPTER 8

Teens and Drowsy Driving

When school let out on June 1, 2015, sixteen-year-old George Sinclair was ready for a nap. A student at San Diego's St. Augustine High School, he was exhausted after having stayed up most of the previous night studying for finals.

When he woke up, though, he wasn't in his bed—he was still in the front seat of his pickup truck, where he'd narrowly missed being impaled by a fence post. Sinclair had nodded off while driving and rolled his truck off the road and into a wooden fence. Although the post had punched through the windshield and right through the steering wheel, Sinclair had shifted just enough as the truck slid so the post ended up under his armpit.[153]

THE SCOPE OF DROWSY DRIVING

Despite the striking details of Sinclair's near miss, the circumstances that led to it were hardly unique.

In a 2017 report, "Asleep at the Wheel," the National Highway Traffic Safety Administration (NHTSA) noted that drowsy driving is considered a factor in about 7 percent of all crashes and about 16.5 percent of all fatal crashes, which would have equated to about six thousand drowsy-driving deaths in 2016. (The report also noted some researchers consider this an underestimate and would place the total at more than eight thousand.)[154]

It's hard to pin down the exact number, given that state databases don't list drowsy-driving crashes in a separate category. The designation is also a subjective one: there's no Breathalyzer equivalent that can be administered on-site the way there is for drunk driving.

Instead, it's up to motorists, their passengers, or other observers to report that the driver was tired and/or fell asleep—feedback that can't always be obtained, especially in the case of fatalities.

Nevertheless, in a study released in 2018, video footage of more than 3,500 drivers showed the number of crashes involving drowsiness was close to 10 percent.[155]

For that study, footage had been gathered over the course of several months using in-car video cameras. Researchers analyzed the footage from the three minutes preceding each crash—captured at a rate of fifteen frames per second—so they could measure the proportion of time drivers had their eyes open vs. closed.

"You can see it with your own eyes on the video," Brian Tefft, a senior researcher with the AAA Foundation for Traffic Safety and one of the study's coauthors, told me.

"When someone's falling asleep, you'll see their eyelids slowly drooping," he explained. "When we look at measures like that . . . we know that the overall proportion of crashes that involve moderate to severe fatigue or drowsiness is in the vicinity of 10 percent or more."

Tefft compared the effects of drowsy driving to those caused by driving under the influence of alcohol. "It's not a perfect comparison, but I think it's a pretty solid [one]," he said.

In another study of Tefft's, using data from the US Department of Transportation, he found the crash risk for drivers who'd slept less than four hours the previous night was roughly equivalent to having a blood-alcohol concentration level of .12, which is well over the .08 legal limit in the United States.[156]

For drivers who'd gotten between four and five hours of sleep, the risk was about the same as having a blood-alcohol concentration level of .05, still a significant level of impairment. Along with the state of Utah, "most other developed countries around the world have a blood-alcohol limit of .05 or lower," Tefft pointed out.

Unlike driving under the influence, however, the risks of drowsy driving aren't always as readily recognized or heeded. "It doesn't start off with the same stigma of being intoxicated," he noted.

Even more worrisome, fatigued motorists are more likely than drunk ones to get behind the wheel *even though they know they're impaired.* According to a AAA Foundation for Traffic Safety report released in 2020, 24 percent of respondents said they'd driven at least once in the past thirty days "while being so tired that they had a hard time keeping their eyes open!" Another unsettling statistic: 10 percent said they'd driven at least once after having consumed "enough alcohol that you thought you might be over the legal limit."[157]

So, why is this so widespread? In addition to Tefft's observation about the relative level of stigma, the fact that drivers were significantly less worried about being pulled over for drowsy driving compared to drunk driving (per the same study) probably factored in too. It's also possible drivers simply overestimated their ability to keep themselves focused and awake, choosing to power through despite knowing they were fatigued.

Even when drivers don't actually nod off behind the wheel, there are still a number of ways fatigue creeps in.

Driving requires split-second decision-making and responsiveness, both of which are impaired by drowsiness. Even moderate sleep impairment has consequences: In his analysis of data from the Department of Transportation, Tefft found drivers who'd slept for five or six hours were more prone to what he called the "simple lapses in attention" all drivers experience periodically, such as failing to notice a traffic signal or misjudging how much time it takes to clear an intersection.

"They made the same kinds of mistakes that we all make from time to time," Tefft said, "but they made them more often."

More severe than lapses in attention are what are termed "microsleeps," which may last for less than a second but can have serious ramifications. Not only is the vehicle still moving, but "a lot can change in the traffic environment," Tefft said. There's also an additional time lag while the driver reorients to the situation, further slowing response time.

And then there's outright falling asleep, which means (obviously) the driver simply isn't responding at all. "For all intents and purposes," Tefft said, "you've relinquished control of the vehicle."

Tefft found that the drivers who'd slept less than four hours and then caused a crash were the most likely to report having fallen asleep. Severely sleep-impaired drivers were also more likely to have lost control of the vehicle or shown signs of overcompensating (for example, oversteering to try to correct drifting out of their lane), which could suggest they'd had a microsleep and were trying to recover from it.

Major drowsy-driving crashes make headlines every few years, such as the truck that crashed into actor Tracy Morgan's limousine in 2014. But curbing drowsy driving remains an ongoing challenge, especially when it comes to noncommercial drivers.

To date, only two states, Arkansas and New Jersey, have laws in place about driving while fatigued. The New Jersey law, passed in 2003, was the first in the nation. It's called Maggie's Law, in memory of a college student killed in 1997 by a driver who hadn't slept in thirty hours.

TEENS ARE ALREADY DANGEROUS BEHIND THE WHEEL

Teen drivers are risky enough even without layering in lack of sleep. They're more likely to crash than drivers in all other age groups, and that risk is highest during the first month after they obtain a license.[158]

In fact, data compiled by the CDC show that in 2018, vehicle crashes were *the leading cause* of injury and death for fifteen-to-twenty-four-year-olds.[159] That same year, there were 4,492 people killed by young drivers (defined as up to age twenty by the NHTSA): a combination of the teens themselves, their passengers, and those they crashed into. An estimated 199,000 teen drivers were injured in crashes that same year, according to NHTSA data.[160]

That's due to a confluence of factors.

First, teen drivers simply aren't as experienced as more-seasoned drivers. Most states only require about fifty hours of supervised driving before getting a license, which is still a far different scenario than when a teen actually gets behind the wheel without an adult copilot. And some states don't require any supervised driving hours at all.

As new drivers, teens aren't yet adept at recognizing various situations and knowing how to respond quickly and appropriately, whether it's gauging the amount of time to get through an intersection once the light turns yellow or deciding whether they should brake or swerve to avoid hitting a squirrel.

They're also likely to be distracted while driving. According to data released by AAA in 2020, more than a third of teen drivers said they'd texted while driving at least once in the past thirty days. And nearly as many confessed to running a red light at least once during the same timeframe![161]

Teens are also less likely to use seat belts, as drivers or as passengers.[162]

These behaviors exemplify what's known about teens' judgment (which is often lacking) and their penchant for risk-taking—both hallmarks of the teen brain, as we saw in earlier chapters.

The brain remodeling in process during the teen years means impulsivity and reward seeking have already revved up, while executive functioning lags behind. Teen drivers are functioning without the benefit of a mature prefrontal cortex, and are making decisions accordingly, all while behind the wheel of a fast-moving vehicle that weighs three thousand pounds or more.

Fortunately, every state now has graduated driver-licensing requirements in place which help counter the risks posed by teen drivers. The specifics vary, but most states require a set number of hours of supervised driving before getting a license and place restrictions on underage passengers and late-night driving. Teens are issued a restricted license specifying these conditions and generally can't apply for an unrestricted license until they turn eighteen.[163]

In addition to setting limits during the peak risk-taking years, these requirements help ensure teens acquire enough initial experience while they're still supervised so they'll be safer drivers once they're on their own.

Graduated licensing requirements have been effective in reducing teen crashes since the mid-1990s, when they first began to be broadly implemented.[164] Still, there's only so much they can do to curtail dangerous teen behavior: one 2013 study revealed teens had applied makeup, changed their clothes or shoes, and even done homework while they were driving![165]

SLEEPY TEENS ARE EVEN MORE DANGEROUS

So, what happens when these same teens are operating a vehicle while they're running on fumes?

Nothing good, obviously. Teen brains already don't process information at optimal speed, and when they're sleep-deprived, this declines even further.

For teens, lack of sleep "really interacts with lack of experience," Tefft said. "It's going to be all the worse for a young person whose driving skills aren't quite there yet, who's less familiar with some of the hazards they may face on the road, and whose responses to those hazards haven't become quite as automatic as more experienced drivers.' "

Researchers have also shown that as teens' sleep declines, their risky driving behaviors increase, whether it's sending texts or emails or driving without wearing a seatbelt (which was three times as likely for teens who'd slept less than six hours compared to those who'd slept at least eight hours, according to a 2018 research letter published in *JAMA Pediatrics*).[166]

Sleep-deprived teens also react more impulsively to perceived threats[167] and become angry more quickly,[168] as we saw in earlier chapters. Neither bodes well when teens are faced with an aggressive driver, such as someone who tries to cut in front of them.

Finally, teens simply may not have a good handle on how exhausted they are. In an Australian study, researchers found that when teens' sleep was restricted, they performed progressively worse on tasks requiring sustained focus. This was true even for teens limited to seven and a half hours' sleep—an amount that passes for normal for many teens—but was even worse for the more sleep-deprived teens. Both scenarios have worrisome implications for an attention-heavy activity like driving, given that teens may downplay how sleepy they are.[169]

That's what happened to George Sinclair, the teen from San Diego who was nearly impaled by a fence post. He knew he was exhausted but figured he'd be OK since it was just a short drive home. "If you think you're falling asleep, pull over," he said the following day. "Call your parents—they'll come get you."

Why Later Start Times Help

In the wake of the success of graduated driver-licensing requirements, Tefft and other experts view later school start times as the next major policy change that can make a real difference in reducing teen crashes.

Robert Foss, director emeritus of the Center for the Study of Young Drivers at the University of North Carolina at Chapel Hill, has spent the bulk of his career focused on driver safety and teen drivers in particular. He noted the causal effect between changing school start times and teen crashes, with the bulk of the reduction taking place in the afternoon.

"Basically, you shrink the amount of time teens are out there driving, and less driving equates to fewer crashes," he told me.

As for why that's in the afternoon rather than in the early-morning hours, more driving, and therefore more crashes, take place in the after-school timeframe, Tefft pointed out.

In a recent study, Foss found that crashes declined by 14 percent after Forsyth County, North Carolina, shifted its start time from 7:30 a.m. to 8:45 a.m. Afternoon crashes shifted later, reflecting the later ending time for school, but also showed an overall decrease.[170]

The study only included sixteen- and seventeen-year-olds and looked at crashes on school days (rather than including summer, holidays, and weekends) in order to better home in on the effect of the change in school hours, Foss said.

While the specifics vary, a number of other studies around the United States have yielded similar results.

As part of a three-year, multistate study, Kyla Wahlstrom, the pioneering educational researcher from the University of Minnesota, looked at teen crash rates in Jackson Hole, Wyoming. She found there was an astounding 70 percent drop after the local high school moved its start from 7:35 a.m. to 8:55 a.m. in 2012.[171]

Wahlstrom, who called the decrease in crashes "remarkable," noted that the economic and ethnic diversity in Jackson Hole allowed for excellent comparisons to crash data from other urban and suburban student populations. "Although there may be an assumption that this is an affluent area, in fact, many of the students are the children of service workers at local hotels and ski resorts," she said.

Moreover, Jackson Hole High School and an alternative high school were the only high schools within a radius of about a hundred miles, she noted, making it much easier to assess the correlation with the later start time.

Other studies have looked at crash rates for students at high schools with different start times. One 2014 study compared student drivers from a Virginia county where high school started at 8:45 a.m. and students from an adjacent one where school began at 7:20 a.m. Although the two counties had similar demographics, teen crash rates (but not adult rates) were higher in the earlier-starting district over the course of two years.[172]

"When you're trying to reduce crashes . . . you need policies that apply to large groups of people and have the potential to alter their behavior in a beneficial way," Foss explained.

He views later school start times as exactly that type of policy. "Change the [start] time," he summed up, "and you're going to reduce crashes."

RAISING AWARENESS

Drowsy driving has long been part of AAA's driver's education curriculum but has recently been expanded, William Van Tassel, who heads AAA's driver training programs, told me. One new component is a two-week sleep log that students complete, and there are also quizzes on aspects ranging from "highway hypnosis" to various ineffective strategies for combating drowsiness (such as trying to "tough it out" or cranking up the music). There's even a section on the importance of sleep, along with strategies for getting a good night's slumber. Another AAA recommendation: taking breaks while driving. ("Generally every two hours, or every hundred minutes, whichever is more useful," Van Tassel said.) If drivers are really fatigued, the best remedy is pulling over for a rest or a brief nap.

Kathi Wright, a Tennessee-based advocate for teen-driver safety, echoes that advice. In 2002, her seventeen-year-old nephew, Kyle Kiihnl, was walking on the sidewalk near his home when a truck jumped the curb and plowed into him. The driver, a fellow classmate at Germantown's Houston High School, had fallen asleep at the wheel.

Kiihnl died instantly.

Wright now travels around the state presenting to groups of teens about drowsy driving, working with the Tennessee Highway Safety Office and others. She started by calling up a local driving school and offering to present to the teens. "It was a little fifteen-minute talk, and I felt like they were totally blown away with what I had told them, like they had never heard anything [about it before]," she said.

"At the end, I always ask, 'Has anyone had a friend or family member involved in a drowsy-driving crash?' and there are always hands."

The teen driver who killed Wright's nephew hadn't been drinking or using drugs, but he was out late on a weekend night—a known risk factor for teen crashes (which is why many states now restrict teen nighttime driving). It was 2:00 a.m., and the driver was returning home from a concert he'd attended with a church group.

He was driving at a time when he normally would have been asleep in bed, Wright pointed out.

The type of crash that killed Kiihnl—one that occurred late at night and is considered a "run-off road crash"—is more likely when young drivers don't get enough sleep on the weekends, according to a 2013 study published in *JAMA Pediatrics*.[173] That study of young, newly licensed drivers, conducted in Australia, showed that drivers who'd gotten less than six hours of sleep on weekend nights had the highest increased risk between 8:00 p.m. and 6:00 a.m.

"Driving at night is just more difficult," Tefft observed. "It tends to be more dangerous than driving during the day for anybody, regardless of age, but especially so for teens."

Although compliance with teen nighttime driving restrictions is "far from perfect," he said, the laws have had a dramatic influence simply by reducing the number of teen drivers on the road during the highest risk timeframe.

As for Wright, she intends to keep spreading the word about drowsy driving and her nephew's death in the hopes no other family has to experience a similar loss. "By telling his story," she said, "we keep his memory alive."

TEEN-SLEEP TAKEAWAYS

- Driving while drowsy is dangerous! It's an issue for all drivers, not just teens.

- Because teen drivers lack the experience and judgment of more experienced drivers, they're already considered more dangerous on the road. Drowsy driving amplifies this.

- Toughing it out or downplaying the risk doesn't make it any less dangerous.

- Drivers who haven't gotten enough sleep are more likely to make judgment errors, react more slowly, or have microsleeps.

- Later school start times have been shown to reduce teen crashes.

CHAPTER 9

Not All Teens Sleep the Same: Why Sex and Gender, Orientation, Race and Ethnicity, and Socioeconomic Status Matter

Throughout this book, we've generally looked at teens as an overall group, focusing on a broad range that includes middle and high schoolers.

However, teens *aren't* one large monolithic group. Anyone who's spent any amount of time with kids and teens knows a fourteen-year-old is vastly different from an eighteen-year-old. Generally speaking, a fourteen-year-old's sleep needs will be on the higher end of the recommended eight-to-ten-hour range, while an older teen's will be on the lower end.

Beyond age, though, there are a number of additional factors affecting sleep. As we'll see in this chapter, some teens are at increased risk based on who they are and where they live. Further complicating matters, there are often areas of overlap, which create cumulative effects.

Being aware these sleep disparities exist is an important first step. In some cases, if any of the aspects covered here are relevant for your teen, building in additional time for sleep can help address the shortfall. It's also important to recognize getting enough sleep can help provide a buffer for resiliency (as covered later in this chapter).

SEX AND GENDER
DIFFERENCES IN SLEEP

We already know teens shift to later sleep schedules during puberty (as noted in Chapter 1), and for girls this tends to happen at a younger age.

In addition to this timing difference, there are also important differences in the *way* girls sleep compared to boys. Some of these appear to be biologically based, while others appear to stem from one's gender identity.

It's a "paradox," Fiona Baker, director of the Human Sleep Research Program at SRI International (formerly the Stanford Research Institute), told me. Teenage girls and women wake less during the night and get more deep, slow-wave sleep than their male counterparts, but they're **also more prone to insomnia**, which emerges during puberty.

Baker's lab has conducted numerous studies looking into biologically based sex differences, including examining how female reproductive events, including menstruation, affect sleep.

In one study, she and her colleagues found that girls take longer to fall asleep (which, when especially prolonged, is a characteristic of insomnia). The girls would drift off for about thirty seconds, then wake up, then drift off again before truly being asleep (or reaching a state of what's termed "consolidated sleep"). The boys went through this same process, but for a shorter overall timeframe.[174]

The teens were also asked to rate whether they felt worried, tense, or otherwise distracted prior to falling asleep. This, too, was more pronounced in the girls.

In another SRI study, researchers found differences in how being stressed before bedtime affects sleep. (The mere fact of sleeping in a laboratory rather than one's bed is known to be a source of stress, allowing sleep technicians to measure this "first-night stress effect," Massimiliano de Zambotti, the lead author of the study, told me.)[175]

Both boys and girls woke more and took longer to fall asleep on the first night. But only the girls had higher heart rates while sleeping, he said—another characteristic of insomnia.

For girls, "after puberty, the risk for insomnia starts to increase," Baker explained. "Girls are at greater risk for having problems with their sleep, meaning they have trouble falling asleep, and they have trouble with waking up at night and not being able to go back to sleep. That's just more common in girls."

Girls' sleep is also often impacted by their monthly menstrual cycles, especially if they start at a younger age or have painful periods or other symptoms such as premenstrual syndrome (PMS).

As you might expect, when Baker studied young women (ages eighteen to thirty), those who had painful menstruation slept worse when they had menstrual cramps.

The same is true for teens, given that up to 93 percent of teen girls experience menstrual cramps ranging from mild to quite painful.[176] One study of more than five thousand menstruating adolescent girls in China found that one in four reported having moderate or severe period pain. Moreover, severe period pain was linked to insomnia symptoms and poor sleep quality.[177]

The same study also found girls who began menstruating at or before age eleven were more likely to have insomnia in their early teen years. (And eleven isn't even considered particularly young: about one-quarter of US girls get their first period by then, and about half do before age twelve, according to a 2020 report by the US Department of Health and Human Services.)[178]

Additional studies by Baker and others have found that young women affected by premenstrual syndrome, which includes moodiness, also have worse sleep quality and more daytime sleepiness than those who don't experience these symptoms. That's not surprising, given the relationship between sleep and mood, as covered in Chapter 4.

Finally, frequency and duration of periods also matter. One study from South Korea found that adolescent females with irregular periods got less sleep than their more regular counterparts.[179] In Japan, meanwhile, female college students whose sleep was more inconsistent (measured by comparing weeknight and weekend sleep) were more likely to report having severe menstrual symptoms.[180]

Overall, Baker believes **menstruation-related effects on sleep aren't always given as much attention as they should be.** "Even with women and girls who don't have painful menstruation . . . or severe PMS, there's still a good number who will say that their sleep is altered," she said, and that's particularly the case just before they get their periods and during their periods. "There's a lot more complexity with sleep because of the reproductive cycle."

Online Stressors

We'll look at technology (including social media) in Chapter 12, but it's worth noting here that girls may be disproportionately affected.

When a girl sees something upsetting on social media, for example, she may reach out to a friend to discuss and dissect it. "Look[ing] at the broadest gender strokes," said clinical psychologist Lisa Damour, "the general rule is boys are more likely to distract themselves" when they're upset, while girls are more likely to seek out social support.

Although emotional connection is important, "All that talking can actually keep a problem alive and make it feel worse," said Damour, the author of *Under Pressure* and *Untangled*. Girls are also more likely to ruminate, she said, which in turn can impact sleep.

Moreover, internal research released in 2021 highlighted that Instagram use may make some girls feel worse about themselves. As Devorah Heitner, author of *Screenwise*, has written, "Social media can turn up the dial on self-doubt, feelings of exclusion, or worries about physical appearance."[181]

Finally, it's important to note that many girls experience online abuse and harassment. When the humanitarian and girls' rights group Plan International asked more than 14,000 girls in twenty-two countries about their experiences online, they found nearly six in ten respondents had been the target of abusive or insulting language. Even worse, four out of ten had been threatened online with sexual violence. Overall, close to 40 percent of respondents said being harassed online was a source of mental or emotional stress for them or for other girls they knew.[182]

Falling in Love

Even the simple act of falling in love can disrupt sleep—and more so for girls than for boys. In a study of Finnish teenagers, Liisa Kuula, a researcher with Sleep Helsinki at the University of Finland, found girls' sleep was more affected, both in terms of total sleep time and the quality of their sleep.[183]

Boys were less likely to report being in a romantic relationship, but the ones who were didn't have their sleep affected as strongly (although those who said they were in love were more depressed and anxious than their peers).

As Kuula and her coauthors wrote, their findings "suggest being in a relationship is a further disruptor of sleep in adolescent girls." (Of note, the study didn't ask whether the girls were in love with a same-sex or opposite-sex partner, but Kuula believes the sleep disruptions at the beginning stages of a relationship attributable to falling in love would be similar. If anything, girls in same-sex relationships may have higher levels of anxiety, she said, due to potential additional stressors related to their sexual identity.)

WHAT ABOUT SEXUAL ORIENTATION?

Although research is still emerging, studies show that sexual- and gender-minority teens and adults sleep worse than their counterparts. (A note about terminology: "sexual and gender minority" and "LGBTQ+" are both often used as umbrella terms, although some studies have used subsets such as "LGBT.")

This has implications for a larger percentage of teens compared to older generations. In 2020, Gallup surveyed US adults and found 16 percent of the Generation Z respondents (in this case, those who were eighteen to twenty-three years old) identified as lesbian, gay, bisexual, transgender, or other. This was the largest percentage for all age groups, with millennials a distant second at 9 percent.[184]

When the CDC asked high schoolers about their sexual identity as part of the 2019 national Youth Risk Behavior Survey, 2.5 percent identified as gay or lesbian, an additional 8.7 percent identified as bisexual, and 4.5 percent said they were "unsure." The teens who stated they were gay, lesbian, or bisexual slept worse than their counterparts, with just 16 percent saying they slept at least eight hours on a typical school night. (By contrast, 22 percent of "unsure" kids and 22.6 percent of heterosexual kids slept eight or more hours.)[185]

Also concerning: The CDC's survey asked respondents whether they'd "felt sad or hopeless" for at least two weeks at some point in the past year. While one-third of the kids who identified as heterosexual said yes, *two-thirds* of kids who were gay, lesbian, or bisexual said this was the case. (The kids who said they were "unsure" were roughly halfway in between.)

Another report, issued in 2018 by the Human Rights Campaign, surveyed 12,000 LGBTQ+ teens and found more than three-fourths of them had felt depressed in the past week. **And practically all of them—95 percent—said they "usually" or "always" have trouble falling asleep.**[186]

The types of stress and discrimination faced by LGBTQ+ teens fall into two main categories, Ryan Watson, an associate professor at the University of Connecticut (and coauthor of the Human Rights Campaign report) told me. There are internal factors, such as guilt or fear about disclosing one's sexual orientation, and then there are external ones, which include everything from family strife to discrimination to bullying by peers. All of these are "above and beyond the normal stressors of adolescence and childhood," Watson said.

While it isn't possible to tease out how each of these specific aspects affects sleep, the net result is **overall, LGBTQ+ teens have additional sources of stress and are also more sleep-deprived.**

A study of 150,000 Chinese teens, for example, found that those who identified as sexual minorities (defined in the study as being attracted to the same sex or to both sexes) got less sleep than their peers, were more likely to sleep poorly, and were also more likely to be bullied at school.[187]

There's another point from the CDC survey worth noting: the kids who indicated they were unsure of how they'd identify their sexuality were a little less likely to get at least eight hours of sleep than the kids who said they were heterosexual, but fared better than those who identified as gay, lesbian, or bisexual.

"Disclosure of sexual orientation is a complex topic," Watson said when we spoke. Kids who are unsure about their sexuality may struggle internally, but may face less external stress and discrimination than they would if they were "out," he explained.

There also appear to be differences among subgroups of the LGBTQ+ community. One review of current studies, published in 2020, noted that bisexual women and transgender individuals report more sleep issues than other sexual and gender minorities.[188]

And then there's overlap not just between sexual and gender identity but with other characteristics including race and social class.

Some researchers have started to examine this intersectionality, looking, for example, at both sexual orientation and racial and ethnic identity. In an abstract presented at the American Public Health Association's 2019 annual meeting, researchers noted that bisexual adults were "particularly likely" to report getting less than seven hours of sleep. This was even more pronounced for Black bisexual women and for Hispanic bisexual adults.[189]

"Knowing more about this intersectionality would be helpful," said the abstract's coauthor, Charlotte Patterson, a psychology professor at the University of Virginia. "We really just need more research, certainly on sexual minority issues and teen sleep."

RACE AND ETHNICITY
AND DISCRIMINATION

Numerous studies have found **teens of color are disproportionately likely to sleep poorly.** As with sexual- and gender-minority research, however, the categorizations aren't always uniform.

The CDC's 2019 national Youth Risk Behavior Survey provides data for students who consider themselves White, Black, or Hispanic, but doesn't provide any insight into other ethnic groups (including teens who view themselves as biracial).[190]

What's been termed the "Black-White sleep gap" is well documented: even after accounting for other factors such as neighborhood differences, education levels, and income, on average, Black people get worse sleep than White people do.[191]

To date, though, there have been fewer studies delving into how Asian teens sleep[192]—an omission that's been called out as "troubling."[193] (In the CDC's 2019 survey, for example, the categories were White, Black or African American, Hispanic or Latino, and Other—a group that included Asian teens as well as those who were American Indian or Alaska Native, Native Hawaiian or other Pacific Islander, or multiracial but non-Hispanic.)[194]

Nevertheless, a study of Asian, Black, Latino, and White children (ages six to twelve) in New York City found Asian kids got the least sleep of any of the groups (twenty-three minutes less per night than White children, who got the most sleep).[195]

These sleep differences are frequently rooted in discrimination, research shows: one 2020 study found teens who experienced discrimination had more trouble falling asleep that night and felt sleepier the following day.[196]

Recently, I spoke with Tiffany Yip, who chairs the psychology department at Fordham University and was the lead author for both of those studies. Yip has spent considerable time looking at the effects of discrimination on teens' sleep. Interestingly, she's found teens who are still exploring their ethnic or racial identity seem to be even *more* affected by discrimination. As she and her coauthors documented in 2020, when teens who didn't feel a strong sense of connection to a racial/ethnic group experienced discrimination, the effects on their sleep were more pronounced (compared to teens who already identified as part of a racial/ethnic group).[197]

"Being the target of discrimination for being a member of a group that you're not quite sure about yet is especially negative," Yip told me.

By contrast, for teens who felt a strong level of commitment to their racial/ethnic group, this sense of belonging helped buffer them from discrimination-related effects on their sleep.

That's not to say discrimination didn't have an impact: numerous studies have found it contributes to longer-term sleep and mental-health issues.

A 2020 study of adults in the greater Detroit area, which noted that more-severe insomnia is more common among racial and ethnic minorities, found that discrimination was an important driver.[198]

Discrimination has also been associated with a decrease in stage three sleep,[199] which has worrisome implications: not only is this the deepest stage of sleep, as described in Chapter 1, it's essential for retaining and synthesizing new information.

Being Well Rested Helps

When teens do get enough sleep, it can serve as an emotional buffer against the effects of discrimination, as noted in Chapter 4. Specifically, when kids slept better, Yip told me, they "were better able to cope with . . . discrimination-related stress the following day."

How Discrimination Impacts Sleep

The various ways discrimination harms health, including sleep, are complex and the subject of widespread, ongoing research. As a very broad overview, however, it's important to note there are both short- and long-term aspects.

SHORT-TERM

This includes everyday experiences of racism and other discrimination, encompassing everything from overt harassment or fears for personal safety to more subtle microaggressions: offhand comments or minor gestures or reactions that reveal underlying attitudes. These "everyday, subtle experiences" may be more minor, but the effect is cumulative.

In a study of US adults published in 2020, researchers at New York University measured both the frequency and the effects of microaggressions. Not only did Black respondents experience them the most, these experiences took a marked emotional toll.[200]

Even though most of the research has focused on adults, a recent meta-analysis found that teens who experienced racial/ethnic discrimination (including both overt instances and microaggressions) were more likely to have depressive symptoms and poor self-esteem, among other negative effects.[201] This was more pronounced for younger teens than for older ones, suggesting not that the discrimination itself decreased, the authors noted, but that the teens simply became more adept at coping with it.

LONG-TERM

In addition to the immediate effects of discrimination—even just one event is considered a "form of acute social stress"[202]—there are longer-term consequences, Azizi Seixas, an assistant professor at New York University's Grossman School of Medicine, explained.

Discrimination can raise stress levels to an ongoing state of high alert, he said, activating the sympathetic nervous system in a fight-or-flight response.

But the toll of discrimination doesn't just stem from one's own experiences. It's also rooted in what's been passed down, or what are known as epigenetic factors, he said. These multigenerational health effects of trauma can be long-lasting.

In other words, teens may also be dealing with a legacy of discrimination in addition to what they may be facing in their daily lives.

"Many of these genetic or epigenetic predispositions and risks are historical," Seixas said. "What you pass on to the next generation and what you inherited from the previous generation are absolutely critical."

An Interrelationship

When looking at racial and ethnic differences in sleep, socioeconomic factors often come into play. (According to the American Psychological Association, "The relationship between SES [socioeconomic status], race and ethnicity is intimately intertwined.")[203]

Even so, when researchers have taken these SES factors into account (such as the effects of poverty, or of neighborhood environment), these disparities still exist. A study published in 2020 found that Black respondents weren't just more likely to be sleep-deprived (in this case, to get less than six hours' sleep) than their White counterparts; they also didn't appear to see the same "protective benefit of higher income" that White adults did.[204]

THE EFFECTS OF POVERTY AND NEIGHBORHOOD ENVIRONMENT

Socioeconomic factors have a major impact on teen sleep. As with the other factors in this chapter, there are areas of overlap, given that SES is often intertwined with race. And there are numerous elements under the umbrella term of SES, such as household income, parent education levels, and household and neighborhood environment. (A disclaimer: what follows touches on some of these aspects but is by no means comprehensive.)

There are a number of ways poverty chips away at sleep. It's not that income itself promotes sleep, the authors of one study noted: "Rather, it is what the income buys."[205]

To start, "Kids who are living in lower SES [households] are often living in more crowded living conditions," said Amy Wolfson, a psychology professor at Loyola University Maryland who's studied adolescent sleep since 1994. In addition to more people in the household, this may mean sharing a room with one or more siblings, adding to the noise level and making it harder to maintain consistent sleep patterns.

The household may also be disrupted by parents' work schedules, Wolfson added, particularly if they rotate shifts or have less-stable work.

Hunger

There are also more pressing needs, like hunger. Even pre-pandemic, 2.4 million US households were unable to provide "adequate, nutritious food" for their children at some point during 2019. More troubling, kids in 213,000 households either went hungry or skipped one or more meals during the day due to lack of food.[206] In 2020, the situation was even worse: 2.9 million households with children experienced food insecurity, and 322,000 households reported that kids went hungry or skipped one or more meals.[207]

This, too, harms sleep. As Jason Nagata, an assistant professor of pediatrics at the University of California, San Francisco, explained, "Part of food insecurity is . . . stress or anxiety about being able to get enough food to eat."

In a study published in 2019, he and his coauthors found that food-insecure young adults (defined as worrying about not having enough money to buy food at any point during the past year) had more trouble both falling asleep and staying asleep.[208]

That's in addition to the simple fact that going to bed on an empty stomach makes it harder to sleep. Nagata relayed an anecdote from a different study he conducted on hunger: one respondent said staying busy during the day made it easier to distract himself from his hunger pangs, but at night they were impossible to ignore.

The issue is likely even more acute for teens, Nagata said, given their higher caloric and nutritional needs. And teens who are active need even more—up to 3,200 calories a day for active teenage boys, according to the 2020–25 dietary guidelines issued by the US Department of Agriculture and US Department of Health and Human Services.[209]

The effects of poverty extend to other basic needs too, like housing. In a recent study examining how housing insecurity affects sleep, RAND Corporation researchers found that adults who didn't have enough money to pay their rent or monthly mortgage averaged twenty-two minutes less sleep per night than their peers. Those who had to move due to money issues fared even worse. (Of note: all of the adults surveyed were receiving government assistance and presumably already had money-related stress, so these sleep deficits were above and beyond their existing sleep loss.)[210]

Other Neighborhood Aspects

Then there's the neighborhood itself, including aspects such as neighborhood density, noise, and overall safety. All of these impact sleep in various ways. As Lauren Hale, a professor of family, population, and preventive medicine at the Stony Brook University School of Medicine, has said, "I have never seen a study that hasn't shown a direct association between neighborhood quality and sleep quality."[211]

First, noise levels can make it difficult to fall asleep and *stay* asleep.

Researchers consider this just one aspect of "neighborhood disorder," a measure that also includes crime, safety, and even how tight-knit the neighborhood is. One recent study in Philadelphia found that when respondents reported higher levels of neighborhood disorder (which included aspects such as having problems with neighbors or feeling they didn't watch out for one another), they were also more likely to report sleep issues such as insomnia and feeling they had less control over their sleep.[212]

Another study, in Florida, looked at how much sleep teens got based on how safe they felt in their neighborhoods. The teens who felt safe were more likely to report getting at least seven hours of sleep a night, lead author Ryan Meldrum of Florida International University told me. (Note that seven hours, the measure used in the study, is still much lower than the eight-to-ten-hour range recommended for teens.)[213]

Finally, when looking at neighborhoods, it's important to note that historic poverty plays a role. In California, researchers found kids in areas with long-term neighborhood poverty (based on forty years of US Census data) were far less likely to get enough sleep than their counterparts elsewhere.[214] "Neighborhoods that are consistently impoverished evolve to become worse for sleep," lead author Connor Sheehan, who's now an assistant professor of sociology at Arizona State University, told me, due to all of these types of factors such as safety, noise, and access to food.

To sum up, **when it comes to sleep deprivation, some teens have it even worse than others.** Ryan Watson's observation about LGBTQ+ teens is true more broadly as well: the stressors on these groups are *in addition* to what they already face as teens. And, paradoxically, one of the very things eroded as a result—their sleep—is one of the keys to help them be more resilient.

TEEN-SLEEP TAKEAWAYS

- Teen girls are more prone to insomnia.

- The menstrual cycle can affect sleep, as can online harassment.

- Sexual- and gender-minority teens generally sleep worse than heterosexual teens.

- Teens of color generally sleep worse than their counterparts.

- Especially for teens who experience discrimination, getting enough sleep can provide an emotional buffer.

- Poverty and neighborhood environment can negatively impact sleep.

- Be aware that these additional factors can harm teen sleep. When possible, focus on other ways to help teens get enough sleep (such as later school start times).

PART III

· · · · · · · · · ·

HOW TO HELP
TEENS GET
MORE SLEEP

CHAPTER 10

How to Help Teens Get More Sleep: Daytime Considerations

In far too many cases, teens have to contend with the reality of too-early school start times. (We'll look at how to help change that in Chapters 13 and 14.)

But there are also other aspects to take into consideration. Whether it's ill-timed caffeine use, pulling all-nighters studying for tests, or chatting online until the wee hours, teens may be sabotaging their sleep or, at the very least, making it worse.

Fortunately, there are a number of steps teens can take—and you can, too—to help set them up for healthier and better sleep. In this chapter, we'll cover daytime strategies, and in Chapter 11, we'll look at some nighttime ones.

Be Aware of Sleep Needs

Before we look at sleep strategies, it's important to reiterate the underlying premise: sleep is valuable and essential, and getting enough of it *matters*.

It may be tempting to assume your teen can function well on the same amount of sleep you can, but that's not the case. As noted in Chapter 1, until age eighteen, teens need eight to ten hours of sleep a night.

"Just because they *seem* more like adults doesn't mean they're sleeping like adults yet," Stanford sleep specialist Rafael Pelayo said.

There's another way parents may unwittingly convey counterproductive sleep messages, he explained, and it's one dating back to childhood. Many parents reward younger kids by letting them stay up late, or punish them by sending them to bed early.

Even if this never happened in your house (I admit to letting my kids stay up late at various points, which they considered a treat), your teenagers may view staying up late as a sign of independence. Or, they may shrug off the information about the eight-to-ten-hour range, insisting the recommendations apply to *other* teens, but they themselves are just fine with less.

THE SNOOZE BUTTON ISN'T YOUR FRIEND

Let's start at the beginning of the day when the alarm clock goes off. Often, teens hit the snooze button several times before actually getting out of bed, hoping for a bit of extra sleep.

They're not doing themselves any favors: any additional sleep they gain is fragmented and not restorative.

Typically, the alarm clock will sound during REM sleep, Pelayo told me. When you fall back asleep, part of that additional time is spent making the transition to the REM stage. "You can quickly go from stage one into REM sleep," he said, "but you still have this transition stage to some degree."

This cycle then repeats each time your teen hits the snooze button. To actually gain those additional ten or twenty minutes, your teen would be better off setting the alarm later and not disrupting REM sleep.

As Pelayo summed up, "You're exchanging dream time for non-REM time, which I think is just a bad deal."

It may be your teen hits snooze simply because it's become the pattern. Instead, though, it's better for the alarm to ring closer to the time they actually get up, allowing for a few quiet (awake) minutes in bed.

Or, perhaps waking up feels too impossible the first time the alarm sounds. While a loud alarm clock (eventually) does the trick, it's not pleasant for your teen or for other members of the household.

Start School Later's Ziporyn Snider still recalls the "sonic boom" alarm clock her younger daughter used in high school. "It sound[ed] like an air raid," she told me. "I would wake up really thinking there was an air raid and I'd jump out of bed and run down the hall to her room." Meanwhile, Ziporyn Snider's daughter would still be sound asleep, even as the device was shaking her bed.

A less jarring option: a sunrise alarm clock with a built-in light that gradually brightens to full daylight strength to help coax your teen awake.

LET THERE BE LIGHT

Whether or not they're using sunrise alarm clocks, teens benefit from being exposed to bright light to help them feel more alert.

"I think bright light in the morning upon first waking is really critical," pediatric sleep psychologist Lisa Meltzer said. "It helps you wake up [and] helps get your internal clock on schedule."

This can be as simple as opening the curtains and turning on the lights, she said. But, if it's the depths of winter (or it's still pre-dawn darkness outside), super-drowsy teens may benefit from a light therapy box. While they're more commonly used in treating seasonal affective disorder (SAD), they can also help boost morning alertness.

"For kids with really difficult circadian phase issues, we will often recommend them," Meltzer said, although "turning on the lights is probably sufficient."

CONSIDER A SCHEDULING CHANGE

There may also be adjustments or workarounds for your teen's early morning classes.

Encourage your teen to schedule more engaging classes at the start of the day, Maida Chen, who directs the Sleep Center at Seattle Children's Hospital, suggested. "Something like orchestra or band—it's a little harder to be sleepy through that."

A PE class is another good option, she said, given that being physically active helps boost alertness.

What if the first class of the morning is an academic one? If your teens have the flexibility to choose when they take specific classes, encourage them to do so based on which subjects engage them the most and whether they feel most alert first thing or later in the day.

Annabel Zhao, who graduated from Radnor High School in 2020, said first-period math helped her stay engaged because it was fast-paced. (For her, the early afternoon was when the drowsiness hit.)

Some schools also include study-hall periods in the schedule; if your teen's does, slotting this in for first period can also help.

Look at the timing of athletic practices too, Galit Levi Dunietz, a sleep epidemiologist and assistant professor of neurology at the University of Michigan, suggested. If there are crack-of-dawn or late-night sessions, it's worth considering a different sport or team.

(One bright spot: as awareness of healthy school hours spreads, some schools are expanding this focus to cover extracurriculars as well. In Biddeford, Maine, as noted in Chapter 7, both before-school and late-night practices were banned in 2016 when the high school moved to an 8:30 a.m. start time.)

There's an additional option to consider: online classes. Even if they're not offered by the school, it's worth checking to see if they'll be accepted and will count toward graduation. (I was clued in to this by another parent.) When my son was in high school, he was able to fulfill his art requirement by taking a two-semester class through an online accredited academy. This meant he didn't have a 7:30 a.m. class his senior year and was able to start the school day at 8:30 a.m. instead. The class was asynchronous, enabling him to watch lectures and complete assignments on his own schedule.

Beware of Overscheduling

Academics are just one part of teens' busy days. In addition to class time and homework, most teens are also involved in extracurricular activities and may have jobs or other time commitments too. All of these take time, obviously, but it's easy to underestimate the cumulative impact.

Planning tools can help, said Denise Pope, cofounder of Challenge Success, a nonprofit affiliated with the Stanford Graduate School of Education. One example the group developed is a pie chart that teens can use to estimate how many hours they spend on each activity per day.

There's also a second resource Pope recommends: a worksheet allowing teens to break down their time commitments within each category, such as extracurriculars and homework, in more detail. It's based on one developed by Miramonte High School in Orinda, California, and has space for students to plug in the estimated amount of homework for each class as well as their time commitments for other activities.

Miramonte and some other schools that offer these tools to their students often include school-provided estimates for homework loads by class, Pope noted. However, this type of information can also be gathered by teens themselves simply through informal conversations with other students.

Using planning tools like these can offer a good reality check for teens and their parents about how much time all of these various commitments take up each week. On the worksheet, nine hours per night is already budgeted for sleep so it doesn't get overlooked, Pope said. The worksheet and pie chart are available on Challenge Success' website and are also included in the appendix.

SET REASONABLE EXPECTATIONS

It's also important to acknowledge that heavy course loads and myriad extracurriculars are often fueled by the drive to be successful and get into a "good" college. While these can be a motivator, they can also lead to burnout and exhaustion.

Taylor Ruiz Chiu, profiled in Chapter 4, called the dynamic a "college arms race." Looking back on her high school years, "I just remember feeling like the expectations on me, whether they were self-inflicted, or [from] my parents or my teachers or peers, or just school as an institution, were so oppressive," she said.

With this pressure coming from multiple sources, addressing it takes a multi-pronged approach, as well as a broader mindset.

"Success is not just about grades and test scores," said Pope of Challenge Success. She stresses to parents that having their kids attend top-tier schools won't help them "find meaning in life." She added, "In the long run, you can go to a whole host of colleges and be as successful."

Pope cited numerous studies, including those showing that attending a selective school didn't translate into higher long-term earnings except for first-generation or "traditionally underserved" students.[215]

Nor do graduates of selective schools report higher levels of engagement or satisfaction in their careers. "You can be a slacker at Harvard and not learn as much as someone in community college," she said. "There's no difference in terms of future well-being or job satisfaction."

It's helpful for parents to reassess some of their expectations, Pope added. "We walk [them] through this . . . Is it about the bumper sticker on your car?"

Students, too, have internalized this pressure. In Challenge Success surveys dating back to 2018, **high school students cite their workload as a top source of stress.**[216]

It's even morphed into what Annabel Zhao, the former Radnor High School student, called "misery poker"—complaining about how little sleep you got, only to be bested by another student. "It's this competition of 'Oh, who slept the least?' "

And it comes at a cost. In Singapore, teens average three hours of studying on school nights (and just six and a half hours of sleep), a 2020 study found. Even more concerning: 10 percent of respondents said their homework load topped five hours a night. Those who spent more time studying and less time in bed (which is how sleep time was measured in the study) reported more frequent depression.[217]

"Reducing adolescents' workload outside of class may benefit their sleep, schoolwork-life balance, and mental well-being," the authors concluded.

Also of note: the authors point out that while Singapore is a "hard-driving Confucian-heritage culture" like Korea, Japan, China, Hong Kong, and Taiwan that prizes academic achievement, students at high-performing schools in Western cultures spend similarly long amounts of time on homework each night.

This certainly tracks with what Pope of Challenge Success has seen. "We have kids taking, like, seven APs at a time—it's crazy," she told me. "You're doing double the load of what a college student does. And here's the difference: [high school students] are in school all day; college students have chunks of time in between their classes, [which] don't meet every day."

Some schools are now enacting policies to address student workload and the accompanying stress, such as setting nightly homework limits or capping the number of AP and honors-level classes students can take. At one school Challenge Success has worked with, Beckman High School in Irvine, California, freshmen are limited to two such classes, with one additional class allowed each year.

Also making a difference: a PTA-backed effort to focus on homework quality, rather than sheer quantity. The resolution was passed by the California PTA in 2014 and then by the national PTA, bringing widespread visibility to the issue of the homework volume students face.

There's one final piece that may help lessen the pressure: colleges themselves have made changes to the admissions process, spurred in part by the pandemic. "I would say almost two thousand colleges were test-optional or test-blind [in 2020]," Pope told me, with the change slated to remain in effect for the next three to five years. Even after that, though, she expects many colleges will stay that way (similar to the University of California system, which has permanently eliminated standardized tests as part of the admissions process).

"I would say that in the majority of cases, we're going to see the schools that are test-blind or test-optional keep these policies around for a while. That would be my preference," she said.

Her message to parents: "There's enough stress in your child's life. Use this as a gift and take it off of your child's plate."

THE ART OF THE NAP

If your teen is exhausted, a nap can help. But there are caveats.

First, it's important to recognize that naps are a way to supplement nighttime sleep, not replace it.

Second, the timing matters—a lot.

Why Nap?

Needing a nap on a regular basis is a sign you're not getting enough sleep at night, said RAND Corporation senior behavioral scientist Wendy Troxel.

Given that teens are chronically sleep-deprived, napping can be a necessary strategy, as it is for military members, she said—a telling analogy, given that adolescence shouldn't be as exhausting as serving in a combat zone.

"Our teenagers are not the same as frontline soldiers who may have to, for operational requirements, be sleep-deprived," Troxel said.

(In fact, in an acknowledgment that inadequate sleep drags down performance and well-being, the US Army's 2020 health and fitness manual not only includes an entire chapter on sleep, it encourages soldiers to take periodic naps "to restore wakefulness and promote performance.")[218]

It's also important to remember that naps help compensate for sleep loss but don't fully erase its impact.

In a Singapore study of sleep-deprived teens, researchers evaluated the effectiveness of naps for teens who had gotten no more than five hours of sleep for five nights in a row. One group had the opportunity to take a one-hour nap each afternoon, while a second group had quiet time instead (during which they watched a documentary).[219]

At several points during the day, both groups completed brief tests to assess their attentiveness, working memory, and other functions. Those who napped had a better ability to stay focused than those who didn't, especially as the week wore on, but still fared worse compared to a control group of teens who'd been allowed to sleep up to nine hours each night.

The takeaway isn't just that getting enough sleep at night is the best strategy—not a surprise!—but that naps can help bridge the gap when this doesn't happen.

If you didn't get enough sleep the night before, "Build in a nap," said Chris Winter, author of *The Sleep Solution*.

Know, too, that simply resting can also be beneficial compared to no downtime at all. "Close your eyes for thirty minutes," he said. "If you fall asleep, great. If you don't, there's still a lot of benefit from that."

He added, "You can control resting [but] you can't control sleeping."

In other words, don't stress out if you can't fall asleep—it isn't going to help make it happen (and may make it *less* likely). Resting may not have the same restorative benefits as actually falling asleep, but it's still a way to get some downtime and a mental reset.

When and How Long?

Nap timing is key, as you might guess.

In general, think of naps earlier in the day as adding to the sleep you missed the night before, Winter said, whereas napping too late in the day takes away from your upcoming sleep at night.

More specifically, "You don't want your [teen] to nap after 3:00 p.m.," the University of Michigan's Galit Levi Dunietz told me, "and you don't want them to nap more than thirty to forty-five minutes." If it's longer than that, they may wake up groggy.

The other concern with naps is that they may end up sabotaging sleep at night, Winter pointed out.

Plus, **if your teen is regularly relying on naps, the new routine may become self-reinforcing.** Especially if the naps are too long, or too late in the day, they can exacerbate the problem and create a vicious cycle, said Troxel.

The bottom line? "If you see that napping is interfering with falling asleep," said Dunietz, "then you shouldn't [nap]."

TIME YOUR CAFFEINE INTAKE

In addition to taking naps, teens often rely on caffeine to cope with their exhaustion.

This makes sense: caffeine is relatively inexpensive, and it's readily available in everything from sugary coffee confections to sodas to energy drinks. And, as noted in Chapter 5, it's a great stimulant.

The issue, though, is it can result in *worse* sleep if teens ingest it too late in the day. (US Army research psychologist Harris Lieberman defined "too late" as after mid-afternoon.)

That's because caffeine use blocks the effectiveness of adenosine, which signals sleepiness. And until the effects of the caffeine wear off, we don't feel the adenosine-driven urge to sleep. It's still there, but essentially masked by the effects of the caffeine.

The amount of time caffeine takes to wear off is surprisingly long. In *Why We Sleep*, neuroscientist Matthew Walker noted that the half-life of caffeine is roughly five to seven hours, which means half of it is still in your system after that amount of time.[220]

That's why, as noted in Chapter 5, **caffeine can create a vicious cycle, making it difficult to fall asleep at night, which then leads to more sleepiness, and more caffeine the following day.**

Caffeine Naps

There is one oddly counterintuitive use of caffeine that may work: a "caffeine nap," which means drinking coffee and then taking a short nap of about twenty minutes right afterward. (It's even recommended on a website for railroaders sponsored by the Federal Railroad Administration.)[221] If done properly, *including at the right time of day*, as noted above, it's considered to be more effective than either strategy alone.[222] You get some restoration from the brief nap, followed by a boost of alertness when the caffeine kicks in. Keep in mind, though, if you do this later in the day, the caffeine may make it harder to fall asleep at night.

GET ACTIVE

Finally, encourage your teen to get enough physical activity during the day. It's good for health for a number of reasons, including its effects on sleep.

Again, research backs this up: specifically, a 2019 study examining teens' physical activity levels and their sleep over the course of a week.[223]

On days when the teens were more active compared to their average levels, they fell asleep earlier and slept longer.

But on days when they were *less* active than average, it was the opposite: they went to sleep later and slept less. (This was also true for teens who spent more time being sedentary than their peers did.)

Specifically, the study measured the amount of time the teens spent doing "moderate-to-vigorous physical activity," the term used by the US Department of Health and Human Services. This included activities like walking, running, playing basketball, or doing aerobic dance.

Being physically active spurs the brain to release more of the hormone that encourages restorative sleep, Stanford's Pelayo noted in *How to Sleep*.[224]

It also boosts mood and can help improve mental health, which is a benefit in and of itself and may also improve sleep.

As a side note, while simply being more active than usual has a positive effect on sleep (as noted above), the guidelines published by the US Department of Health and Human Services call for at least an hour a day of moderate-to-vigorous physical activity for school-age children and adolescents. Unfortunately, less than one-fourth of high schoolers are meeting this guideline, according to the CDC's 2019 national Youth Risk Behavior Survey.[225]

Finally, keep in mind that the time of day for exercise *may* matter, or it may not.

"Identify what works for you," said Cheri Mah, a physician scientist at the University of California, San Francisco, and sleep consultant for numerous sports teams. "I have plenty of athlete [clients] who still sleep well, even exercising prior to bed, or that's just part of their lifestyle because they play late games."

Teens who find it hard to fall asleep after an evening workout should try to minimize them or move them earlier in the day, Mah noted. If that's not possible, she said, "make sure they have a wind-down routine" (something we'll cover in the next chapter).

TEEN-SLEEP TAKEAWAYS

- Don't hit the snooze button—it's not an effective way to squeeze in additional sleep.

- Bright light first thing in the morning boosts alertness.

- When scheduling classes and activities, don't forget to factor in sleep.

- Be strategic about naps and about caffeine.

- Being physically active during the day can make it easier to fall asleep at night.

CHAPTER 11

Other Ways to Help Teens Get More Sleep: Night Moves

What time your teen goes to bed matters, but there are also other considerations.

The following evening strategies can help promote a good night's sleep. (For information about technology, see Chapter 12.)

TIME YOUR STUDYING

Does your teen wait until the last minute to start homework or projects? There are many valid reasons (including being overscheduled), but the result, all too often, is not getting to bed until the wee hours.

Schools themselves may inadvertently encourage this behavior by setting late-night deadlines for electronic submissions of assignments: when the deadline is 11:59 p.m., it's tempting to plan accordingly.

But late-night, last-minute studying actually isn't effective.

"There's not a lot worse than an all-nighter for anything that involves memorization or computation," neurologist Chris Winter pointed out.

That's because getting a good night's sleep helps ensure knowledge actually gets retained. As Matthew Walker wrote in *Why We Sleep*, sleep after learning "effectively clicks the 'save' button on those newly created files."[226]

In a study conducted in Singapore, researchers assessed teens' recall of GRE-type vocabulary words by having them learn new information in cram sessions. During the cram sessions, the teens learned five new words a day for four days in a row (twenty words total). This was compared with a non-cram scenario: learning and practicing all twenty words daily over the same timeframe (but for the same total amount of study time).

Then, the researchers upped the ante even further by restricting the teens to just five hours in bed per night to see how this affected their recall.[227]

Interestingly, *all* of the students (the sleep-deprived ones and the well-rested ones) performed similarly when they'd learned and reviewed the words over the four-day period.

With the cram sessions, though, it was a different story: the students who'd gotten only five hours' sleep fared worse than their well-slept counterparts.

In other words, sleep deprivation plus cramming is a double whammy. As the authors noted, "Vocabulary learning is especially impaired when poor study strategies are combined with insufficient sleep."

These results suggest that for sleep-deprived teens, a strategy of **learning and reviewing information over the course of several days is more effective than cram sessions.** (Regardless, though, five hours in bed is nowhere near enough time for teens!)

Avoid the Last-Minute Crunch

Denise Pope of Challenge Success suggests parents review assignments with teens and help them divide the work into separate steps. Ideally, the teacher will be doing this, she noted, perhaps by setting interim due dates for rough drafts. That said, "It's an appropriate role for parents to take if the school is not doing that."

A recent study of college students underscored that getting better sleep throughout the learning timeframe yields dividends. Students taking an introductory chemistry class at the Massachusetts Institute of Technology wore Fitbits for an entire semester, providing researchers with insights into their sleep over several months.[228]

It turned out that just getting enough sleep the night before midterms wasn't enough to make a difference. Instead, **the students who'd slept well (meaning both sleep duration and quality) the entire prior month got higher scores.**

As one of the study's authors summed up when the results were released, "It's the sleep you get during the days when learning is happening that matter[s] most."

BE CONSISTENT

When it comes to sleep, getting on a good schedule is a far better strategy than relying on weekend sleep to make up the shortfall.

For starters, the latter probably isn't even realistic. Let's say your teen is averaging six hours a night during the week. Even using the lower end of the eight-to-ten-hour recommendation, that's a two-hour deficit each night. With ten hours to make up by the time the weekend rolls around, your teen would need to sleep thirteen hours both nights (the recommended eight-hour minimum, plus an additional five).

You can't really make it up later, UCLA's Adriana Galván pointed out. "Think of it like food," she said. "You wouldn't be able to just say, 'Oh, I'll just eat on the weekend and make up for it.' "

The other issue with bouncing between marathon sleep sessions on the weekend and short nights during the week is that it's akin to jet lag. When your sleep oscillates that much, you're dealing with a similar mismatch known as "social jet lag," Galván said.

The reality, too, is the catch-up sleep your teen gets on the weekend is really only a stopgap measure. In the Singapore nap study cited in the previous chapter, the researchers also looked at whether "recovery" sleep on the weekends (when the students could sleep up to nine hours) reversed the effects of their sleep loss the previous week.[229]

Sadly, it did not.

When tested on sustained attention, the teens improved, but not to the baseline levels they'd had before undergoing five nights of just five hours' sleep. Even worse, the following week, when participants went back to getting five hours of sleep (to mimic another school week of inadequate sleep), they continued to perform progressively worse on the tests. In other words, the two nights of catch-up sleep were like a Band-Aid that masked the lingering sleep deficit but didn't resolve it.

These results track with those of the MIT study mentioned earlier in this chapter, which found that students whose sleep fluctuated dramatically over the course of the semester had worse end-of-semester grades than their peers who kept more consistent hours.

Even more important, inconsistent sleep has worrying mental-health implications.

In one study published in 2021, researchers tracked the sleep patterns of first-year medical residents for an entire year using Fitbits. As you might guess, the residents who got the least sleep had more depressive symptoms. Even more striking, though, residents whose sleep schedules bounced around the most had more depressive symptoms.[230]

So, what's the best strategy if your teen isn't getting enough sleep on school nights? Chris Winter, author of *The Sleep Solution*, shared his thoughts with me.

"Instead of thinking about your [teen] needing eight hours of sleep a night, think of them as needing fifty-six hours a week." Looking at total sleep over the course of a week and building in smaller fixes throughout the week are better than saving it all up, he said.

And if catch-up sleep *does* need to happen on the weekend, there's a way to get it that's less disruptive: encourage your teen to get up close to their regular wake-up time and then take a nap later on. "That way," he explained, "you've kept your schedule intact, versus getting up at one o'clock in the afternoon."

FOCUS ON WINDING DOWN

Have a Bedtime Routine

Do you remember your child's early years? When your teen was a baby, you probably had a nighttime routine—perhaps even an elaborate one—to encourage him or her to sleep through the night. That bedtime routine may have morphed during the toddler years to include a book or other nightly ritual and continued to evolve over the years before you finally extricated yourself from the process.

It's time, now, for a new routine—specifically, helping your teen come up with one they can do on their own to prime themselves for sleep.

Being intentional about winding down for the night can be powerful, I was told by UCSF physician scientist Cheri Mah, who regularly recommends it to the professional athletes she works with "as a way to transition from [their] crazy schedule into getting themselves prepared to sleep for the night."

With teens, too, "it's all about the routine," pediatric sleep psychologist Lisa Meltzer said. The "same activities, same order, same time, every night make a big difference."

Our brains aren't like computers, with on/off switches, she pointed out. Instead, she recommends thinking of them as having dimmer switches. "It takes them a while to shut down," she explained, "and that bedtime routine gives the brain time to power down."

As for what the routine includes, it's up to the individual, but the most important aspect is that it's *consistent*, Meltzer said.

Try Listening

Listening to an audiobook or podcast is another way to help your teen wind down. It "gives the brain just enough to focus," Meltzer explained.

Some of her patients even tune in to a favorite video or TV show, flipping their phones over so they're listening but not watching. "The idea is that it's just the audio," she said, which helps "quiet their brains."

Dim All the Lights

Another consideration is the overall lighting in your home.

In a recent study published in *Nature*, researchers measured evening light levels in participants' homes and the effect on their circadian systems. They found that homes with energy-efficient lights, which typically emit more blue light than traditional incandescent bulbs, had more of an impact on melatonin levels.[231]

The results also showed that individual sensitivity to light varied quite a bit. That said, though, "The average home would suppress melatonin by nearly 50 percent in the average person," the authors concluded.

Why this matters: melatonin is what primes us for bedtime. If the timing of when this hormone is released is delayed, our sensation of sleepiness is also delayed.

An easy step Galit Levi Dunietz of the University of Michigan recommends is turning down the lights in the house at night. "After 10:00 p.m., I dim all the rooms," she told me.

Another option teens may find appealing is red or orange mood lighting in their rooms, which is considered less likely to affect melatonin and more conducive for sleep.[232]

In Chapter 12, you'll find advice about blue-blockers and other ways to lessen the blue light backlit screens emit. (You'll also learn why blue light *isn't* considered the primary issue with nighttime screen use.)

Think Pink

Both light and sound can be characterized by color. Light contains the entire rainbow of wavelengths from shortest (blue/violet) to longest (red). Sound is also classified by waves, with different frequencies associated with various colors. Just as white light contains all colors of the spectrum, white noise contains all the audible frequencies.

Pink noise is often preferred for sleep and relaxation, as is pink or red light (at the other end of the spectrum from the blue light that boosts alertness).

Bring on the Noise

You're probably already familiar with white noise, a hissing static-y sound containing all of the frequencies of sound. It's similar to white light in that it contains the entire spectrum, and it can mask disruptions that could otherwise disrupt sleep.

Because of this, though, white noise isn't always the best for slumber, New York University's Azizi Seixas told me. "If the volume is turned up, it really is quite distracting."

So, what's better than white noise?

Pink noise, according to Seixas. "It essentially suppresses the volume of the higher frequencies, so what you're getting is a much more mellow emission of noise." (And if you're wondering what pink sounds like, it's more akin to water in nature—the susurring rhythm of waves on the beach, or the patter of rain.)[233]

Other colors can also be relaxing, such as brown noise, which sounds "more like a rumble," Seixas said.

In his own household, he's found brown noise helps his young child wind down in the evenings. "Especially for bedtime, when he might be kind of amped . . . it centers him."

Take a Bath

A lengthier wind-down routine might also include a relaxing bath—something the US Army now recommends for its soldiers. In addition to encouraging naps, as noted in the previous chapter, the Army's 2020 health and fitness manual suggests "taking a warm shower or bath" to "facilitate the transition to sleep."[234]

Whether it's warm or hot is certainly up to personal preference, but, as Matthew Walker wrote in *Why We Sleep*, a hot bath is a way to relax, plus "the drop in body temperature after getting out of the bath may help you feel sleepy."[235]

DON'T RELY ON MEDICATION

It's tempting to turn to supplements or prescription remedies, but the sleep experts I spoke to generally aren't fans.

Perhaps the most commonly used is melatonin, which is widely available and relatively inexpensive. It's classified as a dietary supplement, which means it's far less regulated than either prescription or over-the-counter medications. As a result, "You don't know what you're getting," Meltzer said—a worrisome prospect, given that you're supplementing a hormone that plays a critical role in regulating your body's rhythms.

Among the issues she and others cited: melatonin levels in various products can vary significantly, and there may be other undisclosed ingredients as well.

"My preference is that kids don't use it," Meltzer said. "For the general teen, I don't think it's necessary."

When it comes to prescription sleep medication for teens, neurologist Chris Winter takes a similarly dim view. "Show me one study that shows [it's] . . . going to improve sleep quality or even duration significantly," he said.

FURRY FRIENDS

Our family dog snores—a lot! Even though she's a source of comfort, her presence in any of the bedrooms at night would be quite a distraction. It turns out, though, not everyone feels the same way (or perhaps they have quieter pets). Recently, researchers in Canada looked into the effects co-sleeping with a pet had on adolescent sleep. A third of the kids in the study (who ranged from eleven to seventeen) said their pet slept with them at least some of the time. Compared to the other respondents, they slept just as well, and just as long, overall. In fact, the kids who frequently co-slept with their pets rated their sleep quality as higher.[236]

So, while it may seem that a pet in the bed would be disruptive, if Fido's presence is soothing to your teen, the mental-health benefit seems to outweigh this. My takeaway: if your teens like having a pet in the room (or even in the bed) and don't think doing so harms their sleep, don't worry about it.

An App for Teens

Doze (DozeApp.ca) is a free app specifically designed to help teens improve their sleep.

First, teens use the app to track their sleep for two weeks (including what time they got in bed, what time they actually started trying to fall asleep and how long it took, whether they woke during the night, and what time they finally woke and then got up the next morning). This information is crucial for an accurate assessment, Colleen Carney, director of the Sleep and Depression Laboratory at Ryerson University in Toronto, told me.

Based on what teens provide through the sleep diaries and brief quizzes, the app prompts them to set realistic goals and offers targeted tips.

Carney, who developed Doze, described it as providing evidence-based treatment in a format designed by teens—everything from the overall mood and feel to how the information is presented. One result: the app allows users to set their own goals. The teens "basically did not want to be told what to do," Carney said.

Doze also uses motivational interviewing techniques to help pinpoint what the teens see as their main priority, which may not always be their nightly sleep. If, for example, they're most concerned about feeling sluggish during the day, the information will be framed accordingly. "That's fine," Carney said. "Working on daytime goals will [still] help with sleep."

Another teen-friendly feature: the information is presented in bite-size chunks. "No matter how much text we gave them, the teens always said less, less, less. Everything had to be distilled in brief little sound bites." Teens can choose to keep clicking through if they're seeking more details, Carney explained, plus, the quizzes they complete were designed to "lead you sneakily through the information." There's also a companion workbook available through the site.

WHEN TO SEEK HELP

Should your teen see a sleep specialist? If your teen wakes "feeling unrefreshed" despite getting the recommended number of hours, or has chronic insomnia (defined as having trouble falling asleep and/or staying asleep for three or more nights a week for at least three months), a consultation may be in order, said Stanford clinical professor Rafael Pelayo, who specializes in treating sleep disorders.

In addition to assessing the quality of your teen's sleep, the specialist will screen for sleep disorders. It's important, though, that your teen be on board. "As a sleep doctor, the first question I ask is, 'Whose idea was it for you to come here today?'" Pelayo said. "Because most of the disorders we're dealing with in regard to adolescence are circadian disorders, and the principles of treating them involve the motivation of the person to change the behavior."

In a teen with delayed circadian rhythm disorder, the internal clock may run on an even later schedule than what's already expected in adolescence—for example, being unable to fall asleep until about 1:00 a.m.

There are also sleep-related breathing disorders, a category ranging from snoring to obstructive sleep apnea (which means breathing actually stops and starts during sleep). In that scenario, "No matter how much sleep they get, they're going to be tired," Pelayo said.

Another possible cause is restless leg syndrome, which may make it difficult to fall asleep and may also impair sleep quality.

Typically, the first step is a screening by your teen's primary care provider, who may then refer you to a sleep specialist. However, as Pelayo wrote in *How to Sleep*, "If your sleep complaints persist and your doctor doesn't take the problem seriously, it's time to seek out a sleep-medicine physician."[237]

PAY ATTENTION TO YOUR OWN ROLE (AND YOUR SLEEP)

As a parent, you may find negotiating bedtimes and setting new guidelines (perhaps for tech use) make things *more* stressful—the opposite of the calming wind-down period you envisioned.

Try to choose a more neutral time for these discussions rather than during the evening, when your teen may already be feeling stressed.

Remember, too, a sleep-deprived teen is likely to be more prickly. In a study of parent-teen interactions, the kids who'd slept better reported fewer arguments with their parents, Nancy Sin, an assistant professor of psychology at the University of British Columbia, told me.

And finally, don't neglect your own sleep. Aim to be a role model by following the same advice you're giving your teen. Not only will it strengthen the message, it will help set the stage for better interactions.

If you're regularly getting less than seven hours' sleep, you're likely not functioning at your best, including as a parent. (And when your fuse is shorter *and* you're dealing with a sleep-deprived teen, the outcome likely isn't a good one.)

"When kids are well rested and when parents are well rested," clinical psychologist Lisa Damour summed up, "everything seems to go better."

TEEN-SLEEP TAKEAWAYS

- Waiting until the last minute to study doesn't just harm sleep; it's also not effective. Planning ahead is a better strategy.

- Keeping a consistent sleep schedule beats playing catch-up on weekends.

- Teens benefit from a wind-down routine before bed. Try podcasts, dim lighting, soothing noise, and/or a warm bath. And pets in bed are just fine.

- Generally not recommended: supplements and prescription medication.

- If sleep issues persist, consider having your teen screened for other contributing causes.

- Being well rested is important for parents too!

CHAPTER 12

What about Tech?

No book about sleep (much less teen sleep) would be complete without looking at technology and social media.

Unlike those of us who *do* remember the "before" times, our teens are digital natives. These technologies have always permeated their lives.

When the Pew Research Center surveyed US teens in 2018, 95 percent of them said they have access to a smartphone. And 45 percent said they're online "almost constantly"![238]

What's more, they're often "screen stacking," using multiple devices at once. A 2021 study of eight hundred teenage girls found that two-thirds of respondents did so on weeknights, and **more than a third said they were on at least two devices in bed at night.**[239]

HOW TECHNOLOGY AND SOCIAL MEDIA AFFECT TEEN SLEEP

Teens' tech use affects their sleep in three ways:[240]

- The time they spend online (or watching TV) cuts into their sleep time
- The content itself is stimulating and engaging
- The light emitted by the devices delays when their bodies release melatonin

The first one seems pretty straightforward: staying up until 2:00 a.m. scrolling through social media or playing a video game cuts into sleep time.

In fact, studies have shown teens who don't use their devices in bed get more sleep than those who do.

In 2016, a meta-analysis of previous studies of more than 125,000 kids found that those who used portable media devices (such as smartphones) before bed were less likely to get enough sleep—and their sleep quality was worse.[241]

So, why do teens do it? Refer back to item two: What they're doing is stimulating and engaging.

Social Media

Social media has what Jennifer Shapka, a developmental psychologist and professor at the University of British Columbia, calls a "baked-in, addictive quality." And it's immersive by design.

(A 2017 TED talk by former Google design ethicist Tristan Harris and the subsequent 2020 documentary, *The Social Dilemma*, give relatively brief, very unsettling overviews of this.)

"Part of the functionality of social media apps," Shapka recently wrote, "is that they provide alerts, notifications or 'likes' that are designed to draw our attention to our devices to let us know that a pleasurable award awaits."[242] We quickly become conditioned by these cues.

Like Rats Seeking Food

As a study published in 2021 found, the compulsion to use social media is akin to that of rats seeking food. In lab experiments with rats using a Skinner box (essentially, an enclosed box to measure animal behavior based on specific cues), the rats quickly learned that certain actions, such as pressing a lever, resulted in a food reward.

When we use social media, there's a similar process of reward learning at play, the authors noted. After analyzing more than a million posts on Instagram and elsewhere, they found "likes" affected both when and how often users posted.

In other words, **for social media users, "likes," rather than food, are the reward.**[243]

This penchant for reward-seeking is true for all of us, but even more so for teens, given that their brains are primed for it.

However, even though teens are wired to seek out rewards, their impulse control hasn't yet kicked in, as we saw in previous chapters. As a result, they're even more responsive than adults to the deliberately enticing world that awaits them online.

Unfortunately, what they encounter online isn't always rewarding.

"It's an emotional slot machine," clinical psychologist Lisa Damour said, borrowing an analogy Harris uses. "You just don't know what you're getting."

Sometimes, you'll find "this funny, charming, delightful . . . thing that you wanted to see right before you went to bed," Damour explained. When that happens, "You got what you came for."

Other times, though, "You pull the arm of the slot machine and you get something you didn't want to see, or wish you hadn't seen."

This dynamic can easily create emotional havoc for teens. And, it can be even more disruptive for girls, given their proclivity for rumination, said Damour, the author of *Under Pressure*. (Refer back to Chapter 9 for more about online stressors for girls.)

Factor in the heightened odds girls face of online harassment, and the emotional and mental-health repercussions are even more apparent: a recent global survey by humanitarian and girls' rights group Plan International showed that 58 percent of girls have been harassed or abused on social media. Of these, the vast majority reported multiple types of harassment—everything from body shaming to threats of sexual violence.[244]

Online Gaming

Like social media, online games are also designed to maximize engagement. Completing a mission or quest or "leveling up," for example, can easily take far more time than the user intended to spend online.

"Game developers often use token economies and variable reinforcement schedules," Shapka explained in a 2019 paper. These aren't just known to be "highly motivating," she wrote; they're also "very effective at shaping our behavior."[245]

In 2011, in the name of science, seventeen Australian teenage boys volunteered to play a fast-paced violent video game before bed and then let researchers record their sleep. The teens, who were already regular gamers, played for fifty minutes (considered a "normal" amount) on one night, and for two and a half hours on another night.[246]

Unsurprisingly, playing for two and a half hours resulted in less sleep. And even after gaming that long, the teens said they wanted to play more!

Of note, the teens in the study were playing a solitary video game, not a massively multiplayer online role-playing game (MMORPG). These types of multiplayer games, such as *World of Warcraft*, have been linked to poor sleep quality.[247]

A related concern: **internet and video game addiction can harm teen sleep.**

While estimates vary, one 2020 study of more than six thousand Chinese teens and young adults, all of whom were gamers, found that 17 percent met the criteria for internet gaming disorder, a proposed psychiatric disorder that includes symptoms such as an inability to quit or reduce time playing, continuing to game despite problems, and hiding the extent of the issue.[248]

Television and Binge-Watching

Watching TV is more passive than gaming or using social media, but the way we do so is quite different than it once was.

With content widely available on demand rather than on a set schedule, there's often no need to wait to view subsequent episodes. This "unprecedented access to television content" has enabled binge-viewing—yet another thief of teen sleep.[249]

In a survey conducted in November 2017 by Deloitte, 91 percent of fourteen-to-twenty-year-olds said they binge-watch TV shows (which they defined as watching six episodes in one sitting)—the highest of all age groups surveyed.[250]

Again, this is encouraged by design. When one episode ends, the next one is programmed to start automatically if the user doesn't take any action. This "seamless episode delivery" encourages increased consumption.[251]

And it's a method that works as it was designed to. In 2015, researchers at the University of Central Florida conducted a series of focus groups with college students to find out more about what motivated binge-watching. Among their findings: the automatic segue to the next episode, including the on-screen countdown to the next episode, is itself an enjoyable part of the experience.[252]

Still, "the vast majority of the participants reported feeling sometimes out of control," the authors wrote, with spontaneous binge-watching taking up much more of their time than they'd intended.

"I just go to Netflix real quick but then it turns into five hours," one student said. "It's like oh my god what time is it?"

It isn't just that binge-watchers are spending more time watching shows than they intended to; they're also more likely to have what researchers term "cognitive pre-sleep arousal."[253] In other words, **they have trouble "turning off their brains" afterward.** And they also have worse overall sleep, as well as more insomnia, as a result.

The Role of Blue Light

In all of these cases, there's a final factor affecting sleep: the blue light these devices emit.

Backlit flat-screen TVs, smartphones, computers, and tablets use LED light because it's efficient and durable. (Plus, LED screens are generally thinner.) However, LED light in the evening exposes us to blue light at a time when it's not helpful.

Blue light itself isn't bad: it's part of the entire spectrum of light, and during the daytime it can boost our mood and make us more alert. But it can be problematic in the evening because it can delay sleep.

There are two ways it does this, according to Michael Grandner, who directs the sleep and health research program at the University of Arizona. First, it "send[s] a daytime signal when you may not want a daytime signal," he explained on the *Sleep Junkies* podcast in 2020. "And the second thing is, it just biologically suppresses melatonin."[254]

Meanwhile, melatonin, the hormone that encourages sleep, is already on a later internal schedule during the teen years, as Mary Carskadon's research showed.

This untimely exposure to blue light (via all of these various backlit devices) can push the timing even later.

REALISTIC ADVICE ABOUT TEEN TECH USE AND SLEEP

Given the multitude of ways using tech devices affects sleep, there isn't a simple or straightforward solution. However, there are some strategies that may help.

Understanding the Lure of Social Media

First, when it comes to social media, it's important to understand that teens are in many ways the perfect audience for its deliberately immersive design.

With its various feedback mechanisms such as "likes," social media interaction functions as "a form of reinforcement learning." As shown in the 2021 experiment comparing our social media activity to that of rats seeking food, the ongoing stream of feedback is a form of reward learning that influences behavior. And teen brains are uniquely primed for this type of reinforcement.

Equally important is understanding how **social media use taps into teens' developmental need for social connection and validation.** It's something we all have, but it's heightened during adolescence.

"We all pay attention to other people's expressions, thoughts, feelings, and opinions of us," Temple University psychologist Laurence Steinberg has written. "Adolescents just do it more than adults do."[255]

And they do so via social media, a platform almost tailor-made to tap into their social needs.

"It's not the technology," clarified developmental psychologist Jennifer Shapka, a professor at the University of British Columbia. "It's what the technology *gets* them. It's their friends; it's their friendship world."

That's echoed by research by Holly Scott and two colleagues at the University of Glasgow, who conducted a series of focus groups with teenagers in Scotland about why they stay on social media deep into the night.[256]

Time online is "an embedded social experience" for teens, the authors noted. And it stems from the same desire for connectedness previous generations of teens expressed through real-life interactions. Crucially, teens view their online activities as an extension of their "real-world" relationships.

Teens' online activity is driven by two primary social motivations.

First, teens worry if they're not online, they'll miss out on jokes and other references that carry over into in-person interactions. **The peak time for this, according to the teens they studied? "Around bedtime when . . . their peers were most active."**

The second (and related) motivation for the teens was meeting the norms and expectations for what they considered to be normal teen social media use.

As the authors noted, the first concern is internally driven (the worry they'd miss out on a shared experience), and the second is externally driven (the teens' desire to meet the expectations others had about when they should be active online).

"There is so much expected social labor not just in posting, but in responding to posts," added *Screenwise* author Devorah Heitner, which can make it almost a full-time job for some teens.

Recognizing these perceived social costs is therefore a key element in addressing late-night technology use.

"Parents need to . . . really understand how important it is [to them]," Shapka told me. Parents may view setting limits as a way to help rein in technology use, she pointed out, but teens see it as an attempt to control their friendships.

There's another risk too, she said: if teens find themselves facing online issues such as harassment, they'll be less likely to come to their parents if they think their parents will respond by limiting their online access.

Advice about Blue Light

Limiting the amount of blue light tech devices emit may help lessen its impact on sleep.

One approach is dimming the brightness of the screen, which reduces the overall intensity of the light; another related option is altering the color display so it skews warmer in the evening. (iPhones, for example, have a "Night Shift" setting with various options for adjusting the brightness and the color.)

Another way to reduce exposure is by paying attention to how close the device is to your eyes. "It's all about how much light is hitting your retina," Michael Grandner explained in a 2020 podcast. "A television on the other side of the room is going to have much less impact than even a relatively dim mobile phone right in front of your face."[257]

When streaming a TV show, for example, watching it on an actual TV is preferable to a tiny phone screen just inches away.

Yet another way to reduce blue-light exposure is through blue-blocking glasses.

The key is getting a pair that's effective, Grandner told me. "If you can see the color blue, [they're] not blocking it."

In several recent studies testing commercially available blue-blocking glasses, he and his coauthors found that red- and orange-tinted lenses performed the best.

The blue-blockers don't need to be expensive to be effective, Grandner said. "If the lenses on your glasses are orange and you're not really seeing much blue or green from them, it doesn't matter if they're a hundred dollars or ten dollars." He recommends blue-blocking glasses rather than a blue-light screen filter, because the glasses also help with other light in the room.

That said, though, **the experts I spoke to don't see the blue light itself as the primary way teens' tech use affects their sleep.**

Grandner told me he thinks the effects of the other two factors (time displacement, and stimulation and engagement) have a bigger impact on sleep than blue light.

To Rafael Pelayo, a clinical professor at Stanford University's School of Medicine who specializes in treating sleep disorders, blue-light filters are like "putting a filter on a cigarette." Yes, the light is important, he explained, "but the issue really is the interaction with the device."

A recent study analyzing college students' social media use provides additional insights. In the study, researchers looked at blue-light exposure and participants' engagement with the content to determine how both factors affected sleep.[258]

Blue-light exposure was assessed both with and without a blue-light filter. To measure engagement with content, researchers had the students view their own Facebook account or a mock account with no photos or friends, and a random assortment of "liked" pages for companies not targeted to their age range (such as Fisher-Price toys). In all of the scenarios, the participants viewed the pages for fifteen to thirty minutes prior to bed.

When the students looked at their own Facebook pages, using a blue-light filter didn't increase their sleep quality. It took both interventions, boring content *and* a blue-light filter, for participants to report a real improvement.

This may be because they were bored with the generic content and only stayed online for the minimum amount required (fifteen minutes), the study authors noted, with this briefer time online therefore having less of an impact. Nevertheless, they wrote, the results suggest " that when viewing social media, filters may not be as effective as sometimes assumed."

Setting Guidelines in the Home

If you're a parent of a teen, you probably already know setting and maintaining clear guidelines about evening tech use is easier said than done.

Most teens need to be online to complete their school assignments. The volume of homework may be keeping them up late, and the nature of that work often requires them to be online.

Helping them plan ahead (as discussed in the previous chapter) can help them manage their assignments so key portions aren't left until the night before.

That said, though, the tricky part can be getting teens to see your suggestions as help, not interference! They're already juggling heavy homework loads and other demands on their time, and being told they need to get it all done sooner may seem like yet one more source of stress.

Moreover, once those assignments are completed, being online is also part of how teens decompress, whether by watching a show or connecting with friends. Technology is an integral part of their social world.

Some experts recommend a hard-line approach: if you pay the cell phone bill, you get to set the limits.

Certainly, you *can* address tech use this way. But should you?

The short answer: probably not. It might be effective, but not necessarily. And it will likely cause other issues.

As kids get older, they get more savvy, Jennifer Shapka pointed out, and their tech use is likely "going to go underground."

The larger issue she sees is that being overly controlling about technology can strain the parent-teen relationship and damage trust. It's better to work *with* your teens to get their buy-in rather than have their tech use devolve into a power struggle.

"It's an evolving relationship," Shapka said. "[Don't] pit yourself against the technology."

LET THEM KNOW YOU RECOGNIZE THEIR WORLD

To start, let them know you understand tech is an important part of their lives and that "your goal isn't just to get the screen away." It's developmentally normal for teens to want more autonomy, and this extends to their tech use too, Shapka pointed out.

SHARE THE RESEARCH AND THE RECOMMENDATIONS

"Base [tech rules] in evidence, not because you're trying to control, but [because] you're trying to help them," Shapka said. "When I tell my kids why I'm making a decision about screen time, I say, 'Here's what the research says.'"

As a starting point, this can be as simple as sharing the three main ways tech use affects teen sleep (from the beginning of this chapter).

As for the official recommendations: per its 2016 policy statement on media use, **the American Academy of Pediatrics recommends not using devices for an hour before bedtime, as well as removing all devices from bedrooms at night.**[259] (The latter point is also important: the 2016 meta-analysis cited at the beginning of this chapter found that access to media devices at night, *even if kids aren't using them*, also negatively affects sleep.[260])

THE SLEEP-DEPRIVED TEEN

LET THEM TAKE THE LEAD

Encourage your teens to try limiting their tech use before bed so they can see the results firsthand, both Shapka and Damour suggested.

Even if they do have their phones in their rooms, there are still ways to minimize the impact. Perhaps, Shapka said, the question is: "Do I sleep better when the phone is plugged in across the room, or when it's right next to me?"

At a minimum, encourage your teens to turn off notifications, which can sabotage sleep (per the box below).

And encourage them to test out whatever the new approach is, even for a week, so they can see the results for themselves.

Tech Use after Lights-Out

Turning off the lights and going to bed doesn't necessarily mean all tech devices have been turned off. In a study of more than 2,300 young adults (undergraduate and graduate students) in Canada, the majority said they used their smartphones and other similar backlit devices every night after they'd turned out the lights. In fact, more than one-fourth of them did so for at least an hour.[261]

Also concerning: nearly one-fourth of the students said their devices woke them up at night at least once a week. When they woke up in the middle of the night, 40 percent of the students got right back on their phones or other devices! (And it's not just Canadians who check their phones during the night: similar results were found in Israel[262] and Malaysia.[263])

START YOUNG

If you've established household tech rules from a young age, it will be easier to enforce them when your kids are teens. Having a "no phones in bedrooms at night" rule in place from the moment your kid gets a phone means you don't have to establish the rule after there's already an issue.

But what if this isn't the case? It's not too late, according to the experts. "It's really about how to work together to figure out what is going to work best for your [teen]," Shapka said.

SETTING (AND EXPLAINING) HOUSE RULES

If you're implementing tech rules for the first time, they won't necessarily be popular. Still, they can be "negotiated as a family, so that people have agency and agree on what they look like," she said.

Again, having evidence and recommendations will be an important part of this discussion, as teens likely won't be excited about the new rules.

And there's another piece to keep in mind, too: you're helping teens establish healthy tech-use habits they can take with them when they leave home, Shapka said. Once they're on their own (without a parent-mandated overnight charging station in the kitchen), they'll need to take responsibility for not letting their tech use sabotage their sleep.

MODEL GOOD BEHAVIOR

If there are household tech rules, you should be following them as well. If all devices are supposed to be charged in a central location such as the kitchen, then that's where your own phone needs to be. And if the rule is no technology in the bedroom an hour before bedtime, you need to follow it too. Unfortunately, this isn't always the case: when the National Sleep

Foundation surveyed families about their technology use in 2014, more than one-fourth of parents said that after going to sleep, they'd woken up at night and then sent or read emails or texts at least once within the past week.[264] That doesn't set a good example, and it certainly doesn't bode well for sleep.

A better approach is being intentional about your own evening tech use and then talking about it with your teens.

"You should be able to say, 'There is a reason why my technology never comes into my own bedroom,'" said clinical psychologist Lisa Damour. And if you're struggling with staying offline before bed, talk about that too, she said.

KEEP IT IN CONTEXT

Some of what's here may be more relevant in certain households than in others; similarly, some of the evidence may resonate more with some teens than others.

"There isn't any one right answer that works for any kid at any moment in their life," Shapka pointed out.

Know, though, that if you're having issues with your teens' tech use, you're not alone—and again, it's developmentally normal.

It's part of "that transition piece where the child is wrestling for control," Shapka explained, "but they're not quite at the self-regulation place or the place where they can be [solely] responsible."

TEEN-SLEEP TAKEAWAYS

- Tech use cuts into sleep.

- Social media is designed to be immersive. It can also create emotional havoc for teens.

- Online gaming and streaming TV also steal time from sleep.

- Exposure to blue light is a secondary consideration.

- Setting tech-use guidelines calls for empathy, patience, and modeling good behaviors.

CHAPTER 13

How to Help Change School Start Times: Strategies for Success

Being intentional about sleep can only do so much. Even if teens were to chuck their smartphones into the electronics recycling bin, it's likely they *still* wouldn't be able to get enough sleep, given how early they have to wake to get to school on time.

As Start School Later cofounder Terra Ziporyn Snider pointed out, "There's only so far you can go as an individual. There have to be some systemic changes too to make a difference."

Poignantly, a study published in 2017 found students at early-starting schools evidently are making an effort to go to bed earlier, but still wind up sleep-deprived. "Despite going to bed significantly earlier than their peers," the authors wrote, "these earlier bed times did not compensate for the time in bed lost in the morning, presumably due to early school start times."[265]

As numerous studies over the years have shown, too-early start times are a main driver of teen sleep deprivation. When schools shift their start times later, teens get more sleep.

It's true in Seattle.

It's true in Jackson Hole, Wyoming.

And it's also true in other countries, such as Singapore, where sleep deprivation is "rampant."[266]

Putting the onus on teens isn't enough. Let's look at how to help bring
about a broader change that's been proven to work: later school start times.

CONNECT WITH OTHERS IN
YOUR COMMUNITY

Getting involved and advocating for change may seem daunting. But you
don't have to go it alone! Nor should you. Coordinating your efforts with
others in your community is more efficient *and* more effective.

"It's really about building a movement," said Christina Holt, who directs
the Community Tool Box, a free online resource offered through the
University of Kansas for bringing about social change.[267] "What one person can do is so much different than what a group of individuals banded
together [with] a common interest can do."

Take the experience of Phyllis Payne, the implementation director for
Start School Later.

Payne started trying to change her district's 7:20 a.m. high school start
time in 2003, raising the issue at PTA meetings. Meanwhile, another
parent had been doing the same at different PTA meetings in their district
in Fairfax County, Virginia, a sprawling area that included about two
hundred schools. A mutual friend said "Hey, you two need to meet each
other," Payne recalled.

From there, the pair reached out to the president of the Fairfax County
Council of PTAs (the umbrella group for the PTAs in the county), who also
supported later school start times. She agreed to run a small item about
school start times in the next issue of the council's newsletter.

"We got four hundred passionate responses with stories about how children and parents had been negatively impacted by early start times," Payne said, "so many that we couldn't respond to each one individually." Their fledgling group, SLEEP in Fairfax, created a website and an online petition to continue raising awareness and building support.

In addition to using social media, the group took every opportunity they could to share information at in-person events. "On back-to-school nights, we would stand outside with flyers," Payne recalled. "We went to football games, sometimes swim meets—any place where parents and students were gathering, we would share information."

They created their own events, too, such as a town hall meeting featuring a sleep doctor, a sports psychiatrist, a student advocate, and a school board member from another district that had already changed its start times. SLEEP in Fairfax also actively recruited volunteers to serve as coordinators at their school sites.

Payne felt comfortable doing public speaking but noted that not everyone was, nor was it a requirement. Those who weren't comfortable doing so volunteered for other roles, like doing background research or looking up sports schedules.

Getting Comfortable Doing Advocacy Work

The Community Tool Box, a free online resource, has guidance on developing your materials, as well as preparing ahead of time, delivering your presentation, and even handling sticky situations during the question-and-answer period.

There's also a comprehensive "Learn a Skill" section covering everything from planning an advocacy campaign to honing specific skills like writing letters to school board members. The tool box, a public service of the Center for Community Health and Development at the University of Kansas, is at ctb.ku.edu.

PTA

As Payne found, joining forces with the PTA was a way to tap into an existing local structure with complementary goals (the health and well-being of students). Not only does the PTA generally hold regular meetings at each school site, it also has a variety of existing communications—Facebook groups, newsletters, email bulletins, and the like—you can leverage to spread the word. Consider bringing up the topic at a meeting, or placing a small write-up in a newsletter to seek out others who want to connect. (Or, like Payne, do both.)

The PTA can also be a powerful advocate for later start times, as it was in California (see Chapter 15 for more information).

"Ask your local PTA to get involved in the issue," said Carol Kocivar, former legislative advocate for the California State PTA and former president of the state organization. And when you do so, she suggests reminding them of the national PTA's support for later school start times. (Their resolution on healthy sleep for adolescents was passed in 2017 and is available on the national PTA site at PTA.org.)[268]

Start School Later

There's a nonprofit group devoted *specifically* to healthy school start times: Start School Later, at StartSchoolLater.net. I reached out to them when I first started writing about the issue in 2016 and subsequently started a local chapter in my community.

The organization started by Terra Ziporyn Snider and Maribel Ibrahim in 2011 has since grown to 136 chapters in thirty-one states and DC (as of the time of this writing), plus chapters in Brazil and Japan. It's a great resource for sample presentations, ongoing updates, and connecting with others doing similar work in their communities. The group also tracks start-time changes around the country and internationally, based on news coverage, and monitors legislative efforts. In many cases, Start School Later is involved in those efforts: The organization co-sponsored the California bill for later start times. Refer to Chapter 15 for more details.

DETERMINE THE SCOPE

Whether you decide to focus your efforts at your local school or at the district or county level will depend on a number of factors, including the size of your community and the way your local districts are organized. In some cases, there may be just one high school in the entire area. In others, like Fairfax County, Virginia, the local high school may be one of many in the district.

Whether there have already been similar efforts may also matter:

- Have start times been shifted in the recent past, even for other reasons, such as transportation budget concerns?
- How were these changes (or attempts) received in the community?
- Have others in your community previously raised the issue of later start times based on the research, and if so, how did it go?

Another key question is how many others are (or are willing to be) involved:

- Are you starting from scratch, or do you envision quickly assembling a larger group?
- As a corollary: Can you identify high-profile supporters, or people who have ties to the decision-makers?
- When thinking about other potential supporters, have you assessed their sphere of influence at the school, regional, or state level? (If they have statewide influence, you may want to look at a statewide effort, as was done in California.)

In short, the approach you take will likely be determined by the circumstances, including your level of resources and support. Know, too, encountering resistance at one level doesn't mean you might not have more success by either narrowing or broadening your sights.

Changing school start times has been done successfully at every level, from just one high school to an entire state, using the various approaches highlighted here and in the following chapter.

DEVELOP A SHARED FRAMEWORK

As those who have successfully changed school start times will tell you, placing the issue within the larger context is critical.

To start, that means providing education about the basics of teen sleep.

It's not just a matter of getting teens to go to bed earlier! Many people aren't aware that this shift to later bedtimes is a standard part of adolescent development.

"When I talk to parent groups, I'll say, 'When your child is a baby and a toddler . . . you read books about this is when they walk, and this is the age when they talk, and this is the age when the first tooth comes in,' " the University of Minnesota's Kyla Wahlstrom told me.

There are developmental milestones for teenagers too, she explains to parents. "With puberty comes the sleep phase shift, the circadian phase delay," she said. "And this is something you should know just as much as you know about your child being a toddler."

Another aspect that's often misunderstood is how much sleep teens actually need.

Through age seventeen, they should still be getting *at least* eight hours a night: the range for teens is eight to ten hours according to the National Sleep Foundation (see Chapter 1 for a chart listing the recommended sleep timeframes by age).

But all too often, teens (and their parents) underestimate their sleep needs.

In one 2017 study, about half of the parents surveyed said they thought seven to seven and a half hours a night was a sufficient amount of sleep for their teens.[269]

Furthermore, the **parents who underestimated their teens' sleep needs were also less likely to support later start times**, the study's lead author, Galit Levi Dunietz, a sleep epidemiologist and assistant professor of neurology at the University of Michigan, told me.

Also noteworthy: "Parents who supported [later starts] were more likely to understand the benefits of sleep," Dunietz said.

Even more striking, the parents who supported the change were four times as likely to believe their kids would get more sleep, and three times more likely to believe they'd do better in school. They were even more likely to see later start times as a way to help reduce their teens' stress levels.

Let's Sleep!

Let's Sleep!, an online educational resource available at LetsSleep.org, has a wide range of short videos and interactive features for students and parents highlighting the ways sleep affects teen health and well-being. Another audience the site addresses is teachers, with a section about integrating sleep education into the health curriculum for each state. The site is an initiative of Start School Later and was developed in conjunction with the Division of Sleep and Circadian Disorders at Brigham and Women's Hospital.

CONNECT WITH YOUR AUDIENCE

Whether you're starting at your individual school or targeting a larger entity such as your district or region, you and your audience have a common goal. At the broadest level, for example, most people would likely agree the goal is to educate the teens in your community in order to help them become productive members of society. This gives you a starting point to show how sleep deprivation is hindering that goal and how later start times can help.

Remember, many of the people you're reaching out to are deeply invested in these students: as parents, as teachers, as employers, or simply as neighbors or fellow community members.

"Focus on what's at stake," said the University of Kansas' Christina Holt, "and why it matters."

Emphasizing the common ground you share is an important starting point, especially if there are areas you disagree on.

Strive to maintain an environment of respect even when there are differences of opinion, Kocivar of the California PTA told me.

"You want to maintain good working relationships," she said. "Even if they're saying things you don't agree with, respond in a respectful way ... 'Have you thought of it this way?' or 'Here's the research we've seen.' Base it on fact and science, rather than emotions, when you're in those kinds of situations."

PRESENT THE FACTS EFFECTIVELY

Payne recommends tracking down local data, if possible, whether at the city, county, or even state level.

In her case, given the size of Fairfax County, her group was able to get a question about teen sleep added to the local version of the national Youth Risk Behavior Survey (the biennial survey conducted by the CDC).

"It helps to have that data," Payne said. "When you see it and it's about your population, then you can't ignore it."

How the numbers are presented also matters: bogging parents and community members down with too many statistics can make it harder for them to see the issue as personally relevant.

"Keep [it] simple," Payne said. "Break it down into the smallest factors. If you can say 'one out of ten,' people understand that better than saying '10 percent.' "

Also important: citing (and even providing) documentation, ranging from the American Academy of Pediatrics' policy statement on school start times to the various studies showing the link between school start times and teen sleep.

LEVERAGE THE EXPERTS

In the ideal scenario, the superintendent or someone else in a similar leadership capacity will be a visible and public supporter of later school start times. But you may not have this (or may not yet know if you will). Even if you do, bringing in local experts can give your efforts a major boost.

Perhaps you're just getting started with making local connections and developing a shared framework about why later start times are important. Is there a local pediatrician or sleep specialist who can join your group, or who's willing to make a presentation at a parent night or a school board meeting?

In San Diego, pathologist Mariah Baughn, a parent in the district, began reaching out to school board members in early 2017, then spoke during the "public comment" section of a February meeting. It took "persistence and phone calls," she told me, but eventually she was able to meet with her board member, who was a child psychologist and was interested in learning more. At every meeting, Baughn wore her white laboratory coat as a visual cue. Another particularly effective technique was a handout she developed showing the overlap between symptoms of mild-to-moderate lead poisoning and chronic sleep deprivation. Lead in the water had been a prominent issue locally, so her handout really caught people's attention.

Maybe there's already some local momentum and visible leadership for later start times. That was the case in Greenwood Village, Colorado, a Denver-area suburb, when pediatric sleep psychologist Lisa Meltzer got involved.

The deputy superintendent of the Cherry Creek School District, who was heading the effort, invited her to present to the board. "I presented the science, I answered questions," Meltzer said. "I'm sure that it helped them justify their decision."

She recalled the deputy superintendent saying that one of the smartest things he did was to partner with National Jewish Health, where Meltzer is a professor of pediatrics. She's continued to be involved in analyzing pre- and post-change data, finding, for example, that even two years after the change, students continued to get significantly more sleep (about thirty minutes more for middle schoolers, and forty-five minutes more for high schoolers).[270]

If you haven't yet gotten senior-level buy-in from your district leadership or the equivalent, you may need to go even bigger. That's what happened in the early stages in Seattle, where Cindy Jatul, who's a high school biology teacher and former nurse practitioner, started mobilizing other parents. The group included Catherine Darley, who's a naturopathic sleep physician and had started a local Start School Later chapter, and University of Washington neurobiologist Horacio de la Iglesia.

Even so, in their first meeting with the district's then superintendent, "He blew us off, pretty much," Jatul said. That's when their group reached out to Maida Chen, who heads the Sleep Center at Seattle Children's Hospital. The hospital is "one of the biggest games not just in town, but in the state," Chen told me. "And we cover five states. So, Seattle Children's has quite a bit of political panache around here."

Start Times Are an Equity Issue

As Stony Brook University's Lauren Hale shared with me, "Sleep deprivation exacerbates preexisting social and economic disadvantage." (For more on this topic, refer back to Chapter 9.)

In Seattle, Cindy Jatul's years in the classroom had made clear to her later start times could help address these sleep disadvantages. She reached out to two prominent local social-justice organizations, the Seattle/King County branch of the NAACP and El Centro de la Raza, whose subsequent endorsements of later school start times were part of the momentum leading up to the Seattle School Board's approval of the change.

In fact, the results of a pre- and post-change analysis, published in 2018, showed that after later start times were implemented, absences and tardies decreased at the economically disadvantaged school in the study. (See "Narrowing the Education Equity Gap" in Chapter 6 for more details.)

SEEK OUT STUDENT VOICES

Hearing from students is a powerful way to personalize the issue and galvanize change.

How those stories are shared may vary: the "Student Hall of Fame" page on Start School Later's website cites everything from bylined local articles to student-produced videos to community presentations.

Some students have taken it even further:

- In Columbia, Missouri, Jilly Dos Santos single-handedly jump-started the change during her high school sophomore year, garnering national coverage. Dos Santos created an online petition, started a student Facebook group, and sent tweets to mobilize students. Her first victory was thwarting the school board's proposal to move high school start times from 7:50 a.m. to 7:20 a.m. Her second: convincing them they should shift to a 9:00 a.m. start instead. "I know . . . it's going to get some pushback," she told the board. "But it is the right decision."[271]

- In Anne Arundel County, Maryland, high school senior Pallas Snider served on the school board—believed to be the only district board in the country where the student member has full voting rights—when later school start times were first brought up for a vote in 2006. (She voted yes.) A couple of years later, her sister, Sage, served in the same role. (Their mother, Terra Ziporyn Snider, founded Start School Later in 2011.)

- In Radnor, Pennsylvania, sophomore Annabel Zhao was recruited for a local committee on adolescent sleep after she responded to an online survey seeking student input. Her involvement quickly ramped up to include doing outreach to other districts, lobbying at the state capitol, and serving on a state advisory committee. By her senior year, her local school board had pushed back the start time by nearly an hour to 8:30 a.m.

- In Sacramento, California, students at a local high school formed a Start School Later chapter in 2018. Their involvement dovetailed with the timing of California's state bill on later start times, which was at that point in the midst of the legislative process. Because of their proximity to the state capitol, the students were able to do in-person lobbying to help educate legislators and their staffs about the issue and share their own personal experiences. They also attended key hearings for the bill to voice their support.

Living on Video

An effective tactic that harnesses teens' technological savvy is using video to document what it's like for teens who are (figuratively) sleepwalking through school. In 2007, Sage Snider, then a junior at Severna Park High School in Maryland (and younger sister of Pallas, noted earlier), made a short film for her media-studies class, as described in Chapter 6. The following year, when she served on the Anne Arundel (Maryland) school board, she shared the film with the other board members.

Another creative take: in Seattle, during the years-long effort for later start times, a group of teens created a short film depicting students as zombies roaming the school halls.

TEEN-SLEEP TAKEAWAYS

- Be strategic and connect with others in your community.

- Seek out resources, such as Start School Later, Let's Sleep!, or your local or regional PTA.

- Providing context and developing a shared framework is key.

- Start times are an equity issue.

- Hearing from local experts can be quite effective, as can hearing from students themselves.

CHAPTER 14

How to Help Change School Start Times: Insights on What to Expect

You've connected with others in your community. You understand the link between later start times and sleep. And you're aware of the many ways teens benefit, from mental health to grades, from athletic performance to driving safety.

In short, you've started the process. Now what?

Especially if you're in an area where schools start too early for teens to get the sleep they need, the situation may seem straightforward: after all, healthy school start times are recommended by the American Academy of Pediatrics and a host of other groups and have been implemented in countless communities.

That said, though, there will be questions. And there will be concerns. There also may be people who are opposed and are quite vocal about it.

This chapter provides an overview of what you're likely to encounter, culled from experiences in communities that have changed their start times and the common themes that emerged.

DON'T RUSH

It's natural to be leery of—or even opposed to—change. Shifting this mindset takes time.

Another key consideration: school schedules impact a range of stakeholders—not just students but parents, teachers, care providers, and more.

In order to identify these, address the various logistical concerns, and get enough people on board, it's critical to avoid speeding through the process.

And, even after this stage is complete, remember that families and others who may be affected will need advance notice so they can modify their plans accordingly.

As the "lessons learned" summary of the 2014 school-start-time-change study specifically called out, **"Adjustments take time."** (The report, produced by Children's National Medical Center on behalf of Fairfax County Public Schools, is a treasure trove of information and best practices from districts around the country.)[272]

Finally, remember that the objections raised (and they *will* be raised!) can be resolved, as they have been in other communities. In many cases, they're "really perceptions of problems," Start School Later's Phyllis Payne pointed out, "rather than actual."

Identifying Stakeholders and Addressing Concerns

In any community, there are "a tremendous number of interlocking pieces," Payne said.

There may be before-school and after-school care providers. There are sports and other extracurriculars, including those outside of school, like club sports or community leagues, which may share practice space. Perhaps there are local businesses, such as tutors, that may be affected, or employers who hire students for part-time jobs.

After you've identified the key stakeholder groups, you'll want to determine which issues are likely to be most relevant so you can be prepared to respond.

Try to identify which groups may be opposed to the change—in many cases, these groups will be stakeholders who are wary of the logistical changes that could result.

Even so, "The perceived challenges tend to be the same from school division to school division," Payne said. "We encourage districts to look for examples of others that have made the change so they can share, 'Okay, you might think that this would happen, but here's what actually happens.' "

COUNTERING OBJECTIONS

The Challenge of Inertia

Perhaps the biggest barrier to changing school start times is a desire to avoid change, coupled with a sense things are fine the way they are.

This is where personal stories come into play, as well as the data about mental health, academic performance, and all of the other teen behaviors covered in this book.

At a high-performing school, for example, it's easy to assume that by extension, the students themselves must be doing well. Sharing some of the data about teen mental health may be particularly relevant in this scenario. Again, if you have information specific to your school or your community, it may have an even greater impact.

There's also a related phenomenon known as omission bias. This means the consequences of *not* taking an action aren't as readily understood as those that arise from making a change. (Start School Later cofounder Terra Ziporyn Snider and two coauthors wrote about this in 2017, in an article about applying behavioral insights when trying to change school start times.)[273] In the case of later start times, it means opponents are readily able to express concerns about how, say, after-school sports will be affected, but don't necessarily grasp the ongoing toll of sleep deprivation on students.

"We tend to overlook or underemphasize what's going on now, and we don't see the harm from doing nothing," Ziporyn Snider explained.

Remember, too, building a base of understanding can be a slow process. "For a lot of people in the community, it's brand-new information," she said. "If you're not living it, if you don't have kids in school or in high school, you don't even think about it. People need to hear and understand that sleep matters."

Along with inertia, challenges often arise about how later start times will affect sports and how they'll impact transportation and family schedules.

Sports

As a starting point, sharing information about the many ways sleep helps athletes can help shift the conversation so it's focused on the *benefits* of the change. (See Chapter 7 for information and inspiration!)

In addition to the positive aspects for athletic performance, it's helpful to emphasize the academic side of the equation as well. Remind parents that getting more sleep impacts grades, which helps athletes maintain their eligibility to play, as noted in Chapter 7.

Logistical issues are often raised too, such as coordinating game times with other schools or needing to address field lighting, Payne pointed out. This is where sharing information about the solutions other schools have come up with can be particularly helpful.

"Sports are often not nearly as difficult to rearrange as people think they might be," she said. Often, practices don't even need to shift later in the afternoon, given that many coaches work elsewhere and need to come to the campus after work.

For those practices that do need to shift slightly later, solutions include sharing field space so it's being used more efficiently, or shaving a bit of time off of practices, Payne said.

A note of caution: be wary of moving practices from after school to before school, which negates the benefits later start times have on sleep.

Some districts have even made the decision to eliminate before-school practices entirely. That's what happened in Biddeford, Maine, when the district changed its high school start times. "If we're doing this, we're going to do it right," Biddeford superintendent Jeremy Ray told me.

Even without this type of policy, though, before-school practices shift correspondingly later when schools move their start times back, which still helps those student athletes sleep in a bit longer.

Transportation-Related Concerns

Transportation is often a perceived stumbling block to changing start times. "There are logistical challenges," Payne acknowledged, but there are also "multiple ways to make it work."

SCHOOL BUS TRANSPORTATION

Not all districts offer bus transportation to school, but those that do often used a tiered system so they can use the same buses for staggered drop-offs and pickups for elementary, middle, and high schools. (More information is in Chapter 2.)

In many cases, those schedules have been in place for quite a while, and it may be time for them to be reevaluated anyway. Because those schedules were generally established before the timing of teen sleep was understood, high schools were usually put in the earliest time slots, with elementary school kids (who actually *do* wake early, based on their body clocks) given the latest pickup times.

Particularly in larger districts, which use multiple buses, transportation planners can use modeling software to come up with alternative schedules. There's also tremendous value in finding out how other similar districts have handled the transportation piece. (Along these lines, Start School Later holds implementation workshops around the country to bring together transportation planners and other stakeholders.)

OTHER WAYS KIDS GET TO SCHOOL

By high school, many students are responsible for getting themselves to school. They may be driving there, catching a ride with a friend, walking, or riding their bike—all of which are more dangerous during the early-morning hours.

Pedestrians and cyclists are harder for drivers to spot when it's still dark out. And student drivers, who are already considered higher risk because of their inexperience, pose even more of a danger when they're sleepy. (Refer back to Chapter 8 on drowsy driving.)

Other Related Family Concerns

The reality for families with kids is that family schedules are often structured around school schedules. Complicating matters, those schedules change as students move up through the school system, with different starting and ending times for elementary, middle, and high schools. (In many cases, kindergartners also have shorter days than other elementary schoolers.)

Parents may already be resigned to having to adjust each time their child switches schools. Nevertheless, it's important to recognize that later high school start times present yet one more scheduling change and provide families with enough advance notice.

Perhaps a district decides to flip its schedule, so elementary schools start earlier and high schools start later. This can end up being beneficial for parents, given that teens, unlike younger children, are generally capable of getting themselves ready and out the door.

In a situation where a parent leaves early for work, teens can also help younger siblings in the morning, if necessary. This can help offset the change in the afternoons for families in which teens may help with care duties. (Another option is for elementary schools to offer additional after-school care, which may be offset by reduced demand for before-school care.)

The bottom line, though, is school schedules *already* don't align with work schedules. The traditional workday doesn't end at the same time the school day does, and that's not even taking into account school-prep holidays, breaks, and summer vacations. (Plus, many parents have jobs with nontraditional hours.) **The stress of having to coordinate various schedules is already an unfortunate reality, and it's not helped in any meaningful way by high school start times that exacerbate teen sleep deprivation.**

Even so, flipping school tiers so elementary schools start first doesn't mean they should start at the crack of dawn, either. A 7:00 a.m. start time is too early for a high schooler, but it's also too early for younger children! (A start time of 8:00 a.m. or later is what Start School Later recommends for elementary schools, with start times of 8:30 a.m. or later for middle and high schools.)

SOME COMMON MISCONCEPTIONS

There are also some concerns that aren't borne out in reality. Here's a quick overview, along with information you can use to address them.

After-School Jobs

If teens get out of school later in the afternoon, won't that harm those who have after-school jobs?

This concern has been raised in many communities but is largely unfounded. In a 2019 study, two research economists at the US Bureau of

Labor Statistics analyzed a nationally representative sample of students at earlier- and later-starting public high schools. They found students at later-starting schools were just as likely to hold down after-school jobs (and spent just as much time at work) as their earlier-starting counterparts.[274]

That's because in most cases, the type of businesses employing teenagers do so in the afternoons and evenings to meet anticipated demand in the after-school and after-work timeframes. A restaurant may staff up for the dinner rush, for example, which isn't affected by what time school ends.

There's also another related consideration: many students who work do so in the evenings and may not get home until late at night. Having a later school start time allows them to sleep in longer in the morning.

Preparation for the Real World

Shouldn't teens get used to being able to function while exhausted? Isn't this good preparation for "the real world"?

No, and no.

Being a student isn't like training for a marathon. **It's not as if getting by on too-little sleep builds endurance.** Kids may get used to feeling exhausted, but they're not gaining anything from the experience.

It's just the opposite. Being sleep-deprived drags down their academic performance, their mental health, their sports performance, their driving ability, and more, as we've already seen. In the best-case scenario, they're functioning well *despite* being exhausted, not because of it.

As for functioning in the real world: work hours can vary widely based on job roles and professions.

Can't Teens Just Go to Bed Earlier?

Having teens go to bed earlier doesn't mean they can fall asleep early (as you already know from reading this far)!

This is why educating community members about the basics of teen sleep is so essential (the "shared framework" discussed in the previous chapter). Not everyone understands that teens' body clocks shift later when they hit adolescence.

As noted in Chapter 1, teen sleep is cut off at the front end by their biology, and at the back end by their schools' required start times. Requiring teens to go to bed at, say, 9:30 p.m. just means they'll stare at the ceiling.

How Do We Know Students Won't Stay Up Later?

There's a wealth of data showing that when schools shift their start times later, students don't just shift their bedtimes accordingly. They actually get more sleep!

In Seattle, the largest city to date to delay its start times (as of this writing), high school students slept thirty-four additional minutes per night. "[That's] a huge increase from a sleep medicine point of view," said University of Washington biology professor Horacio de la Iglesia, who coauthored a study examining the change.[275]

Another study, in Fairfax County, Virginia, found similar results: after high school start times were moved from 7:15 a.m. to 8:10 a.m., students reported thirty minutes' more sleep.[276]

These sleep gains aren't short lived, either. In 2020, *JAMA Pediatrics* published results of a study in the Minneapolis area comparing student sleep at high schools that had shifted to later start times and those that hadn't. Even after two years, students at the later-starting schools got about forty minutes' more sleep. Not only had they *not* shifted to later bedtimes compared to students at the other schools, they also weren't sleeping in as much on weekends (which is a way to assess how much sleep loss they'd built up during the school week).[277]

Teen Tech Use and Sleep

A related concern many raise is that teens are tired because of late-night smartphone use rather than too-early start times.

However, teen sleep deprivation predates smartphones. Long before the iPhone was introduced in 2007, several districts, including Edina and Minneapolis, demonstrated that later start times helped students get more sleep.[278]

Judith Owens, who led the 2014 Children's National Medical Center study commissioned by Fairfax County Public Schools in Virginia, has conducted extensive research examining the impact of the district's 2015 shift to later start times.

In one study, published in 2017, she and her coauthors looked at the use of smartphones and other electronic devices in bed before falling asleep. They found that shifting to later start times didn't significantly impact tech use: students were still using "light-emitting electronic devices" (specifically, televisions, computers, and smartphones) before bed as much as they had previously.[279]

The kids who didn't use their devices before bed got more total sleep than their counterparts across the board, both when school started earlier and when it started later.

However, after start times were pushed back, *both* sets of kids had a net gain of about thirty minutes of sleep on school nights.

The bottom line: despite tech use before bedtime, later school start times are *still* an effective way to help teens get more sleep. That said, tech use is an important consideration as part of the overall mix. See Chapter 12 for more information.

BE PERSISTENT

As noted at the beginning of this chapter, change takes time. That's true even in the best-case scenario where your district or other entity sees the benefits of later start times and is ready to make the shift. But you may find people aren't interested in having the conversation or have already decided it won't work. Don't give up!

If you don't get a response, keep following up. And do the same if you don't get a positive response. Form a group, bring in local health experts (see the previous chapter for inspiration), build awareness by showing up at meetings or starting a Facebook group—whatever makes sense for you. Reach out to others for ideas, including through Start School Later. And keep spreading the word: if one tactic doesn't work, try a different one, such as sharing information about new studies, or forwarding examples of media coverage in a follow-up note. Be attuned to new possibilities as they present themselves.

Refocus the Conversation

This chapter highlights some of the most common concerns that get raised. While it's important to address these and be responsive, **you don't want the emphasis to be on the logistics of the change rather than the rationale for making the change in the first place.** As noted in the previous chapter, developing a shared framework is essential. Not everyone understands the basics of adolescent sleep and the many ways teens benefit from later start times—all of the mental-health effects, academic aspects, behavioral implications, and more, as discussed earlier in the book.

LATER START TIMES AS A PUBLIC HEALTH ISSUE

An essential message to share—and repeat, and emphasize as often as possible—is that **later start times are a public health issue.** That's why the American Academy of Pediatrics released its policy statement in 2014 calling for start times of 8:30 a.m. or later, and why other major medical and public health groups concur.[280]

As RAND Corporation senior behavioral scientist Wendy Troxel has said, "School start times are the only *policy-level issue* that has been identified as directly contributing to the problem."[281]

We've seen in previous chapters that there are a number of steps students (and their families) can take to help counter sleep deprivation. But there's only so much they can do if they're attending schools that start far too early in the morning.

"We cannot treat . . . societal-level problems with only individual-level solutions," Troxel told me. "We need broader-scale, policy-level intervention."

FOR MORE INFORMATION

What's here is just an initial overview; there's a wealth of information available about how various districts around the country have addressed similar issues. See, for example, the 2014 study produced by Children's National Medical Center on behalf of Fairfax County, Virginia, as well as the 2019 report produced by the Pennsylvania Advisory Committee on Later School Start Times at Secondary Schools. These reports, along with individual case studies, are available via the Start School Later website. There's also a section, "Myths and Misconceptions," with more details about addressing concerns.

TEEN-SLEEP TAKEAWAYS

- Change takes time! Don't rush the process.

- Identify the specific concerns and address them.

- Among the issues most likely to be raised are sports, transportation, and family schedules.

- There are several common misconceptions about teen sleep and later school start times, which are addressed in this chapter.

- Teen sleep deprivation is a public health issue.

CHAPTER 15

Later Start Times in California: An Insider's View

The final session of the legislative year is typically a marathon event, filled with last-minute negotiations and drama. Even so, September 13, 2019, stood out for its strangeness.

The school start times bill was just one of hundreds the California State Assembly needed to vote on before adjourning for the year. As the assembly slowly inched its way down the list, our small group of volunteers texted back and forth, anxiously awaiting our bill's turn. We'd been at this stage before, with the bill having made it nearly all the way through the gauntlet, only to be stymied at this final step before reaching the governor's desk.

Suddenly, the proceedings in the assembly were brought to an abrupt halt. The reason soon trickled out on Twitter: in the chamber of the California State Senate, which was working its way through a similarly lengthy list of bills, a protestor in the upstairs gallery had thrown a small cupful of what appeared to be *blood* down onto the senators, yelling, "That's for the dead babies!"

The substance was indeed blood—menstrual blood. And it had splashed onto at least six of the legislators. The protestor, who was quickly arrested, was soon identified as one of the anti-vax protestors who had recently been at the capitol loudly opposing two bills to tighten up exemptions to children's vaccine requirements.

Both chambers were quickly emptied: the senate so it could be investigated as a crime scene, and the assembly as a precaution. During the break, the affected legislators left so they could shower. Both chambers eventually resumed their sessions, but what had already been shaping up to be a long night became even longer.

★ ★ ★

"Menstrualgate," as it was dubbed, was a truly bizarre coda not just to the legislative year, but to the improbable journey I'd set in motion three years earlier, almost to the day, with my September 2016 op-ed for the *Los Angeles Times*. That essay, in which I'd channeled my continued frustration over the early start times at my son's high school, had been the catalyst for SB-328, which was now poised to change start times not just at my local high school, but throughout the entire state.

The topic first hit my radar in the fall of 2015, when my son entered high school. All of our local high schools started at 7:30 a.m. But why? Was this the norm elsewhere, too? As a parent and a journalist, I went into information-gathering mode. Before the end of my son's freshman year, I'd started writing about why schools start so early and the resulting toll this takes on students. I'd also reached out to our district superintendent and gotten zero response.

In the fall of 2016, I wrote about it again, for the *Los Angeles Times*. While the op-ed gave me a boost of local visibility—by then, I'd assembled a group of other parents who also wanted later start times—there wasn't any immediate change. Having recently started up a local chapter of Start School Later after connecting with the group during my research, I shifted my focus to seeing what I could accomplish locally.

Then, in January 2017, I found out my op-ed had sparked something bigger. State Senator Anthony Portantino, whose district in Los Angeles includes Pasadena and surrounding areas, had read it. As it so happened, his daughter's high school was in the midst of assessing whether to move its 7:45 a.m. start time to 8:30 a.m., so he was attuned to both the difficulty of early starts and the rationale for shifting them later. After looking into the issue further, he decided to introduce a state bill about it. His office reached out to Start School Later, which agreed to sponsor the bill and looped in the chapter leaders in the state.

★ ★ ★

The bill, which proposed 8:30 a.m. as the earliest allowed start time for the state's middle and high schools, was introduced in February 2017. From then on, everything kicked into high gear. There had been similar proposed legislation in other states, but nothing of this scope had ever succeeded. And this was California: the most populous state, and one that often serves as a bellwether for other states.

Support and opposition by major groups quickly emerged. The immensely powerful California Teachers Association, along with the California School Boards Association, decried the bill as overreach that impinged on local control. Meanwhile, the California Parent Teachers Association, focused on the bill's merits for kids' well-being, announced its support. The PTA provided key input that helped shape the bill, including suggesting a three-year window to allow enough preparation, as well as clarifying that "zero periods" (optional before-school classes) could still be offered.

Drawing on the legislative experience and guidance from Start School Later, several of us in California formed a virtual team. We were spread across the state: Mariah Baughn (mentioned in Chapter 13) and Beth McNeill in San Diego, me in the Los Angeles area, Irena Keller (who'd founded the statewide Start School Later chapter) in the San Francisco Bay Area, and Joy Wake, Sue Gylling, and Anne Del Core in Sacramento. Another key player: Stanford sleep specialist Rafael Pelayo (who wrote the foreword for this book).

That year, several of us testified at key committee hearings in Sacramento. I jumped in as the de facto communications manager, developing briefing materials and reaching out to education reporters around the state. Wake headed legislative outreach in Sacramento, while Baughn and McNeill were active in San Diego, where several key legislators on various committees were based. Throughout, we kept in regular contact with a growing list of supporters, urging them to send emails to legislators at various critical junctures. And we regularly called on sleep researchers and other experts around the country, whose support was key.

OUR STRATEGIES THE FIRST YEAR

- **"The big book"**: A hefty, bound compilation of research on adolescent sleep and school start times, this was assembled when SB-328 was first introduced, based largely on resources provided by Start School Later, and distributed by Portantino's office to other legislators. It was regularly updated by the Sacramento team over the three-year period.
- **April 2017 school-start-time conference, convened by Start School Later**: In a bit of fortuitous timing, the first national conference on the topic was held two months after SB-328 was introduced. Not only was Portantino a featured speaker, the event was a way to connect with many of the key researchers who would go on to provide support for the bill.
- **Communications outreach**: Fact sheets, media materials, action alerts, and Q&As were essential throughout the process for reaching various audiences, including the media, legislators, and the general community.
- **Support letters**: Our main ongoing message was that too-early start times are a public health issue. As part of this, we kept in regular contact with a large group of medical experts and asked them to send support letters to committee members prior to key hearings.
- **Regular communication with supporters**: Drawing on our own email lists as well as lists of people who had signed a petition

for later school start times, we sent regular updates and encouraged supporters to email committee members prior to key hearings.

- **In-person lobbying**: In San Diego, Baughn and McNeill met in person with representatives at key legislators' offices in advance of committee hearings. In Sacramento, Wake and colleagues held similar meetings, hand-delivered updates to legislators' offices, and arranged for lobbying days involving the entire team.

- **Harnessing new research**: When a major RAND Corporation report detailing the economic benefits of later school start times was released in August 2017, it received widespread coverage. Wake, Gylling, and Del Core ensured the report and highlights of the coverage it received were hand-delivered to every assembly member.

- **Countering misconceptions**: Throughout the entire process, various issues such as the impact on transportation were raised. We addressed these repeatedly, including by providing in-depth analyses of how they'd been addressed elsewhere.

The final hurdle for the bill that year (after wending its way through the senate, then through various committees on the assembly side) was a floor vote by the California State Assembly, where it needed a simple majority of forty-one votes to pass. Leading up to the vote, we knew it would be close. As a political novice, I also learned a lot about the last-minute maneuvering that takes place (as Portantino had joked to me earlier in the year, "There's a lot of politics in politics.")

As it turned out, the vote in September 2017 wasn't even close: just twenty-six of the legislators voted yes, and thirty voted no. The other twenty-three assembly members abstained from voting (which meant they didn't need to take a position on the record).

But Portantino still had another option: he recrafted SB-328 into a two-year bill, providing an extra year for building support. And there was an additional development: in July 2018, he was appointed chair of the

Senate Appropriations Committee, a position that provided more political influence.

Once again, the CTA lobbied hard against SB-328, but this time, at the end of August 2018, the bill got *exactly* the forty-one votes it needed to pass.

All that was needed for the bill to become law was Governor Jerry Brown's signature. Instead, he vetoed it, stating that he believed the decision should be made locally.

The veto was immediately excoriated by the *San Diego Union-Tribune*, which wrote in an editorial: "You can judge a society by how much it values the health of children. For Jerry Brown and much of the California education establishment, what's convenient for adults is what matters, not what's best for children's health. Here's hoping the next governor isn't remotely as callous and anti-science."

NEW YEAR, NEW BILL

With Brown having termed out, 2019 brought a new governor and another chance. On February 15, 2019—nearly two years to the day from when SB-328 was first introduced—Portantino brought it forth again, timing it so it would again be the 328th bill (given that it was already well known as SB-328). There were two new key amendments: an exemption for rural districts in the state, and a start-time change for middle schools to "8:00 a.m. or later" rather than the "8:30 a.m. or later" change for high schools. This provided additional flexibility while still ensuring teens would benefit (given that middle school includes many preteens, while all high schoolers are solidly in the teen years).

This time around, we asked the California PTA to sign on as a cosponsor of the bill. Carol Kocivar, who was the legislative advocate for the state organization, had been convinced of the merits of SB-328 early on, and

Wake worked with her to make the case for official sponsorship. As Kocivar later explained, "We took a really close look at this and asked the most important question: 'What is best for our kids?' "[282] The PTA's sponsorship brought additional visibility and resources, both of which were key. "They were dogged in their advocacy," Portantino noted.

Another major show of support: a letter signed by more than 125 leading medical and public-health experts from around the country. Working with Wake, Terra Ziporyn Snider of Start School Later reached out to the contacts she'd developed over the years, which included many seminal voices in the field of sleep medicine. Again, SB-328 went through the entire process on both the senate and assembly sides. The final stop before reaching Governor Newsom's desk was the floor vote by the California State Assembly—the same hurdle where the bill had faltered in 2017, but which it had subsequently cleared (narrowly) in 2018.

The expert consensus letter was hand-delivered to every assembly member (in fact, it was spotted several times as part of the briefing materials many brought to the floor on the day of the vote).

Then came the final day of the session—September 13, 2019. Given the drama and delay of "Menstrualgate," the vote on SB-328 didn't take place until after midnight (and it wasn't even the last bill on the list). As in 2018, it passed! This time, it even picked up a few more votes than it had the first time around.

There was still one last and formidable step. Governor Gavin Newsom had thirty days to sign it into law—or veto it, as his predecessor had. Unlike Brown, Newsom wasn't known to be an outspoken proponent for local control. (Also, we knew he had four school-aged children, so we hoped he'd be more attuned to the issue of kids needing later start times.)

There was a final blitz of letters to Newsom's office, from organizations ranging from the California Police Chiefs Association (given the public safety ramifications) to the National Sleep Foundation. There were final appeals from supporters including US Representative Zoe Lofgren. And, we knew, there were similar activities opposing the bill underway, with last-minute entreaties from the CTA and other opposing groups urging Newsom to veto the bill.

And there was the endless-seeming wait.

Finally, at about 8:30 p.m. on the *very* last day, Newsom signed the bill. (Unlike Brown, he didn't include a written rationale offering a window into his reasoning.)

WHAT IT FINALLY TOOK: PERSISTENCE, ALLIES, COMMUNICATION, TIMING, AND FLEXIBILITY

During the California legislative journey, these five themes were key to success. (On a personal note, they sum up the trajectory of my own experience as well.) The themes could be seen in the following elements:

- Portantino's expertise at navigating the political process, including the slow build of negotiations, along with fortuitous developments including a change of governor.
- The visibility and endorsement of experts and high-profile allies. This included the California PTA's decision to cosponsor the bill, the consensus letter signed by more than 125 medical and public-health experts, and ongoing support (including letters and calls) from subject-matter experts such as Judith Owens, who'd authored the AAP statement, and Stanford's Pelayo, who testified at every hearing that allowed testimony. US Representative Lofgren, who has championed the issue since 1998 (when she first introduced the Z's to A's Act) made calls to legislators at critical points in the process.

- Extensive communications and consistent messaging, reiterating **that this was a public health issue.** Throughout the process, in stark contrast, groups that opposed the bill characterized start times as something that should be decided locally, in large part because it would preserve local bargaining by key unions. (As Portantino was quoted: "They're not talking about the science or the impact on teens. What they're talking about is the impact on adults.")[283]

- Addressing concerns. As noted earlier in this chapter, logistical issues arise and can be successfully addressed. Being responsive to these was key, and included everything from various bill amendments to one-on-one conversations.

Ultimately, what we were able to accomplish in California drew on the body of research and many efforts to date, as well as on the active support of researchers around the country. May it continue to bolster similar efforts elsewhere.

EPILOGUE

Where We Are Today

Back in 2011, Dr. Mary Carskadon characterized the myriad pressures on teen sleep as "the perfect storm."

Teens' internal cues shift so they're not ready to go to sleep until later at night. They have more reasons to stay up later than they used to, whether it's completing their homework, using social media, or simply not having parents as involved in their bedtime routines. And they generally have to wake up earlier than they used to because of school start times.[284]

When their sleep is squeezed on both ends, she noted, they wind up sleep-deprived.

The metaphor "the perfect storm" also applies to adolescence itself. As we've seen, teens are awash in intense emotions and primed to seek out new experiences. They're feeling increased pressure as academic expectations and other commitments ramp up. And everything they're experiencing takes place against the backdrop of too-little sleep.

It may seem that skimping on sleep is what allows them to get everything else done. But sleep deprivation isn't helping them. It's actually making everything harder.

We've seen what's at stake, and we've also seen there are specific actions to help improve the situation.

It starts with valuing sleep. There are changes we can make in our own households and in our teens' schedules to encourage sleep. From improving nightly routines to reevaluating overall commitments and technology use, there are numerous paths forward.

It means adjusting start times so students don't have to be in school so early. We now know that being awake and alert doesn't just make it easier to learn and retain information; it also leads to a range of academic and other gains. Even high-performing students benefit from being well rested, and their mental health improves too.

At the broader level, it includes addressing the pressure-cooker environment our teens face and taking steps to lower their stress. In their quest to meet all of these expectations, they're short-changing their sleep, and it's harming their well-being. (As neurologist Chris Winter pointed out when we spoke, "Just because you *can* do it doesn't mean you should.")

Already, we've seen some changes: for Fall 2022 admissions, a record number of colleges and universities (about 1,800 as of the time of this writing) aren't requiring students to take the SAT or ACT, according to the National Center for Fair and Open Testing. (Updated information is available at FairTest.org.) And in late 2021, the University of California system announced that it was permanently eliminating the use of standardized tests as part of the admissions process.

Meanwhile, at the high school level, the pivot to remote instruction during the pandemic spurred a number of changes, including later start times. Even after returning to in-person instruction, many schools kept these new start times in place.

"We've seen it in a number of districts all over the country," said Start School Later's Terra Ziporyn Snider, who noted that the pandemic served as a catalyst for many schools that were already considering enacting later start times.

What's more, the new law in California, effective July 1, 2022, means that in the most populous state in the nation, the vast majority of students at public high schools and middle schools—about *three million* kids—will now have healthy start times.

I'm inspired by all of the changes we've seen to date, and hope you are too. May they be a harbinger of even more to come.

Because when teens are well rested, the results are nothing short of transformative.

APPENDIX A

WEBSITES

The following websites (all referenced in the book) are a treasure trove of essential information and helpful resources.

Challenge Success: www.challengesuccess.org
A nonprofit affiliated with the Stanford Graduate School of Education, Challenge Success focuses on redefining traditional measures of student success to help kids achieve better balance and well-being. Its website includes links to the group's white papers and other research, along with numerous other resources.

Community Tool Box: www.ctb.ku.edu
The Community Tool Box is a free, comprehensive resource for bringing about social change. It contains a wealth of information—everything from guidance on getting started to tips for developing materials to advice on handling sticky situations during question-and-answer periods. It's offered as a public service of the Center for Community Health and Development at the University of Kansas.

Doze: www.dozeapp.ca
Doze is a free app designed to help teens improve their sleep. Using the app, teens track their sleep and are then prompted to set realistic goals. Funded by the Canadian Institutes of Health Research, it offers evidence-based treatment in an interactive, teen-friendly format.

Let's Sleep!: www.letssleep.org

Let's Sleep! is an online educational resource featuring videos, interactive activities, and other advice and information for students. The information, which is personalized by state, also includes a section for teachers about integrating sleep education into the health curriculum. An initiative of Start School Later, the site was developed in conjunction with the Division of Sleep and Circadian Disorders at Brigham and Women's Hospital.

PTA: www.pta.org

In 2017, the national PTA passed a resolution on healthy sleep for adolescents (it's listed on the site as a child-health resolution under the "Advocacy" tab). In California, the state PTA's cosponsorship helped bring about the state's school start times law. As noted on its site, the PTA is the oldest and largest child advocacy association in the United States.

Start School Later: www.startschoollater.net

Start School Later has promoted awareness and advocacy for healthy school start times since its inception in 2011. The group cosponsored the California bill for later start times and was a key supporter throughout the process. Its website is a one-stop resource for accessing sample presentations, staying up to date on related news and legislation, and connecting with other like-minded volunteers. One resource mentioned several times in the book, the 2014 school start time report prepared by Children's National Medical Center, can be accessed at StartSchoolLater. net/uploads/9/7/9/6/9796500/blueprint-change-school-start-time-change-reportfinal4-14-14.pdf.

APPENDIX B

PIE CHART/TIME WHEEL

This time wheel, developed by Challenge Success, helps teens look at how many hours they spend on each activity per day.

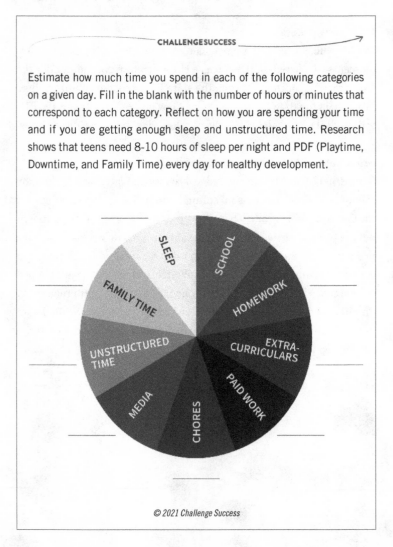

CHALLENGE SUCCESS

Estimate how much time you spend in each of the following categories on a given day. Fill in the blank with the number of hours or minutes that correspond to each category. Reflect on how you are spending your time and if you are getting enough sleep and unstructured time. Research shows that teens need 8-10 hours of sleep per night and PDF (Playtime, Downtime, and Family Time) every day for healthy development.

© 2021 Challenge Success

APPENDIX C

TIME MANAGEMENT WORKSHEET

This worksheet, developed by Challenge Success, allows teens to break down their time commitments within each category (such as extracurriculars and homework) in more detail. Note that nine hours of sleep per night is already included!

CHALLENGE SUCCESS

OVERVIEW

The Time Management Worksheet helps students consider how they will allocate their time for a particular semester/trimester/quarter. Students should estimate hours spent in a 7-day week across the following four categories:

School

The Time Management Worksheet works best when students know the homework load expectations for all of their classes. If this information is not already available to students, we recommend asking every department to complete the worksheet titled "Maximum Homework Estimates" (page 3 of this document). On it, departments can list all classes offered along with the maximum amount of nightly homework students can expect. Page 4 offers an example.

Extracurriculars

This section allows students to capture the structured activities they do outside of school such as sports, theatre, debate, paid work, community service, religious school, outside tutoring, etc. Students should not feel obligated to add an activity to every available line.

© 2019 Challenge Success. Adapted from Miramonte High School's Time Management Worksheet.

Unstructured Time

This section offers a place to list daily activities such as eating, grooming, and chores, as well as time spent outside of school in the following three categories:

Playtime—Time spent doing activities that the student freely chooses to do, such as shooting hoops, playing the piano for fun, hanging out with friends, or reading a book. This does not include scheduled practices or lessons that are captured in the extracurriculars section.

Downtime—Time spent relaxing, reflecting, or just "being."

Family Time—Time when the whole family is engaged in an activity such as eating meals, playing games, hiking, watching a movie, or participating in public service.

Keep in mind that research shows kids need Playtime, Downtime, Family Time (PDF) every day for healthy development. Check out PDF for Teens for tips on how to build more PDF into your week.

Sleep

According to experts, to lead healthy, balanced lives, high school students need 8-10 hours of sleep per night, and middle school students need 9-11 hours. We have pre-populated this worksheet with 9 hours per night. If a student's schedule does not allow for the recommended amount of sleep on most nights, students should consider adjusting their daily or weekly commitments to prioritize sleep.

TIME MANAGEMENT WORKSHEET (CONT.)

Estimate the time you spend engaged in these activities during a typical 7-day week

SCHOOL

TOTAL WEEKLY HOURS: ____

In class time (e.g., 5 days **x** 7 hours = 35 hours)	
Homework: Subject 1*	
Homework: Subject 2	
Homework: Subject 3	
Homework: Subject 4	
Homework: Subject 5	
Homework: Subject 6	
Homework: Subject 7	

EXTRACURRICULARS

TOTAL WEEKLY HOURS: ____

Paid job	
Community Service	
Sports	
Visual & Performing Art	
Non-school assigned homework (e.g., SAT prep)	

UNSTRUCTURED TIME

TOTAL WEEKLY HOURS: ____

Playtime, Downtime, Family Time	
Necessities (e.g., grooming, eating, transportation)	
Chores	

SLEEP

TOTAL WEEKLY HOURS: _63_

Weekday sleep (8-10 hrs/night, says American Academy of Pediatrics)	45 hrs
Weekend sleep	18 hrs

☐ School Total **+** ☐ Extracurriculars Total **+** ☐ Unstructured Time Total **+** [63] Sleep Total **=** ☐ **Your Weekly Total** **

* Ask your teachers to estimate the maximum nightly homework
** 1 week = 168 hours

© 2019 Challenge Success. Adapted from Miramonte High School's Time Management Worksheet.

ACKNOWLEDGMENTS

Bringing a book into the world is no easy feat. It would not have happened without the support of everyone listed here. (I am sure there are others I'll remember to include only after this has gone to press—please know that it was unintentional!)

First, this book owes its existence to Michael Davis, my mentor through the Solutions Journalism Network. (After hearing about my involvement in California's law, my writing, and my passion for the topic, he said, "You should write a book about it!") Michael believed in me and in my ability to write this long before I did, and he's been a sounding board and a key source of moral support ever since. I'm also indebted to the founders of the Solutions Journalism Network, David Bornstein, Tina Rosenberg, and Courtney Martin, along with countless others at SJN, including Allen Arthur, Sara Catania, Jules Hotz, Maurisse Johnson, and Linda Shaw, for your encouragement along the way.

My agent, Joëlle Delbourgo, took me on in the early days of the pandemic and steadfastly navigated the way through the entire publication process. I'm eternally grateful for her kindness, savvy, and perspective.

Thanks to the entire team at Mango Publishing Group, including my supportive editor, Yaddyra Peralta. I know there may be others I've missed, but my heartfelt appreciation to Geena El-Haj, MJ Fievre, Shawn Hoult, Minerve Jean, Brenda Knight, Jermaine Lau, Morgane Leoni, Christina McCall, Chris McKenney, Robin Miller, Hannah Jorstad Paulsen, and Nehemie Pierre.

I am indebted to the entire sleep-research community and your groundbreaking research and insights into teen sleep, school start times, and other related areas. Without you, none of this would exist. Moreover, your expertise, and your generosity in sharing it, are at the core of this book.

(An additional thank-you to the lengthy list of experts I interviewed and quoted throughout!)

I'm also grateful for the tireless efforts and ongoing dedication of everyone involved in Start School Later, including Terra Ziporyn Snider and Phyllis Payne, who were both key resources as I wrote this book, as well as Maribel Ibrahim, Melissa Stanton, Stacy Simera, Debbie Moore, Elinore Boeke, Andra Broadwater, Kari Oakes, and Pallas Ziporyn.

My immense thanks to State Senator Anthony Portantino, who read my op-ed in the *Los Angeles Times*, decided to introduce a bill on healthy school start times, and then expertly shepherded it through a two-and-a-half-year legislative journey. You continue to be an incredible advocate for California's youth.

Carol Kocivar, former legislative advocate for the California PTA, was an early supporter of the bill and was integral to the organization's co-sponsorship. Her advocacy throughout the process and her help since then have been invaluable.

A huge thank-you as well to our small volunteer team in California, especially Joy Wake and Rafael Pelayo. Together with Mariah Baughn, Anne Del Core, Sue Gylling, Irena Keller, and Beth McNeill, we accomplished something incredible. I'm fortunate to have met all of you, and I enjoyed the many, many hours we spent working together!

I'll forever be grateful to the many editors I've worked with, including Susan Matthews at *Slate*, who published my very first article on teen sleep, and Juliet Lapidos, who was formerly the op-ed editor at the *Los Angeles Times*.

I was fortunate to (figuratively) stumble into a supportive writing group right as my book contract was being finalized. Lanier Isom, Ellen Piligian, Laura Westley, and Claire Whitcomb have been my Zoom-based cheerleaders, readers, and sounding boards, offering support and encouragement through the many highs and lows. I'm humbled by your friendship.

There are many other writers, editors, and friends, both IRL and online, who have readily provided advice, encouragement, referrals, and more. Your generosity and wisdom have meant the world to me. I'm sure there are others I'm forgetting, but thank you to Margaret Allen, Chris Beach, Michele Borba, Caitlin Brodnick, Gail Cornwall, Nicole Eredics, Alison Singh Gee, Esther Gulli, Devorah Heitner, Amanda Lewis, Katherine Reynolds Lewis, Matt Lewis, Ashley Merryman, Melinda Wenner Moyer, Ashleigh Renard, Lori Uber-Zak, Tracy Wise, and Allison Williams. And a huge thank-you to Laurel Leigh, whose talent is exceeded only by her generosity of spirit.

Thank you, too, to the Millsians, including Barbara Joan Tiger Bass, Karen Finlay, Misty Hecht, Sian Jones, Heather Kamins, Lee Kaplan, Rachel Leibrock, Jaime Lin-Yu, Mahmud Rahman, Ethel Rohan, Mel Hilario Sattin, Jennifer Soloway, Sarah Stevenson, Tara Weaver, and Sarah Zacharias.

To my close friends and family (you know who you are), my immense gratitude for your love and encouragement. A special shout-out to my sister, Jennifer Newton, who's brilliant and inspiring.

And most of all, to my husband, Josh, and my two kids, Joey and Charlotte. Josh, thank you for always believing in me and being a true partner. I love you with all of my heart. (And the Stephen Ambrose quote is true; every writer should be lucky enough to marry an English major.) And Joey and Charlotte, without both of you, none of this would matter. Being your parent is one of the biggest joys of my life.

INDEX

ENDNOTES

Introduction

1   Danice K. Eaton et al., "Youth Risk Behavior Surveillance—United States, 2007," *Morbidity and Mortality Weekly Report (MMWR)* 57, no. SS04 (June 6, 2008): 1–131.

2   MMWR and Centers for Disease Control and Prevention (CDC), "Reports, Fact Sheets, and Publications | YRBSS | Adolescent and School Health | CDC," August 18, 2021, https://www.cdc.gov/healthyyouth/data/yrbs/reports_factsheet_publications.htm

3   Max Hirshkowitz et al., "National Sleep Foundation's Sleep Time Duration Recommendations: Methodology and Results Summary," *Sleep Health* 1, no. 1 (March 2012): 40–43, https://doi.org/10.1016/j.sleh.2014.12.010.

4   Jessica Lahey, The *Addiction Inoculation: Raising Healthy Kids in a Culture of Dependence* (New York: Harper, 2021), 116.

5   Rafael Pelayo, *7 Tips to Sleeping Well*, TEDxMarinSalon (Video), 2021, https://www.ted.com/talks/rafael_pelayo_7_tips_to_sleeping_well.

Prologue: The Stanford Summer Sleep Camp

6   William C. Dement and Christopher Vaughan, *The Promise of Sleep: A Pioneer in Sleep Medicine Explores the Vital Connection Between Health, Happiness, and a Good Night's Sleep* (New York: Dell, 1999), 58.

7   Mary A. Carskadon, "When Worlds Collide: Adolescent Need for Sleep Versus Societal Demands," *Phi Delta Kappan* 80, no. 5 (January 1999): 348–353.

8   Mary A. Carskadon, Cecilia Vieira, and Christine Acebo, "Association between Puberty and Delayed Phase Preference," *Sleep* 16, no. 3 (May 1993): 258–262, https://doi.org/10.1093/sleep/16.3.258.

Chapter 1: Sleep and the Teenage Brain

9   Elizabeth Kolbert, "Up All Night: The Science of Sleeplessness," *The New Yorker*, March 3, 2013, https://www.newyorker.com/magazine/2013/03/11/up-all-night-2

10   Chip Brown, "The Stubborn Scientist Who Unraveled a Mystery of the Night," *Smithsonian Magazine*, October 2003, https://www.smithsonianmag.com/science-nature/the-stubborn-scientist-who-unraveled-a-mystery-of-the-night-91514538/

11   William C. Dement and Christopher Vaughan, *The Promise of Sleep: A Pioneer in Sleep Medicine Explores the Vital Connection Between Health, Happiness, and a Good Night's Sleep* (New York: Dell, 1999), 33.

12   Ibid., 38.

13   William C Dement and Rafael Pelayo, *Dement's Sleep & Dreams* (Charleston, SC.: CreateSpace Independent Publishing Platform, 2015), 35.

14   Dement and Vaughan, *The Promise of Sleep*, 208.

15 Dement and Pelayo, *Dement's Sleep & Dreams*, 49.

16 Matthew P. Walker, *Why We Sleep: Unlocking the Power of Sleep and Dreams* (New York, NY: Scribner, an imprint of Simon & Schuster, Inc., 2017), 131.

17 Ibid., 127.

18 Ibid., 114.

19 Ibid., 115.

20 Ibid., 53.

21 Stephenie Meyer, "The Story of Twilight & Getting Published," *Stephenie Meyer* (blog), accessed December 3, 2021, https://stepheniemeyer.com/the-story-of-twilight-getting-published/

22 University of Illinois at Chicago, "Growth Hormone Activates Gene Involved In Healing Damaged Tissue," *ScienceDaily*, https://www.sciencedaily.com/releases/2003/12/031204074202.htm

23 Sarah Graham, "Sleep Deprivation Tied to Shifts in Hunger Hormones," *Scientific American*, December 7, 2004, https://www.scientificamerican.com/article/sleep-deprivation-tied-to/

24 Hirshkowitz et al., "National Sleep Foundation's Sleep Time Duration Recommendations." *Sleep Health*. 2015 Mar;1(1):40-43. doi: 10.1016/j.sleh.2014.12.010. Epub 2015 Jan 8. PMID: 29073412.

25 Anne G. Wheaton et al., "Short Sleep Duration Among Middle School and High School Students—United States, 2015," *Morbidity and Mortality Weekly Report (MMWR)* 67, no. 3 (January 28, 2018): 85–90, https://doi.org/10.15585/mmwr.mm6703a1

26 Frances E. Jensen and Amy Ellis Nutt, *The Teenage Brain: A Neuroscientist's Survival Guide to Raising Adolescents and Young Adults* (New York, NY: Harper, 2015), 48.

27 Ibid., 71.

28 Engineering and Medicine National Academies of Sciences, *The Promise of Adolescence: Realizing Opportunity for All Youth*, ed. Richard J. Bonnie, Emily P. Backes, and National Academies of Sciences, Engineer (Washington, District of Columbia) (Washington, DC: The National Academies Press, 2019), 46, https://doi.org/10.17226/25388

29 Walker, *Why We Sleep*, 88–89.

30 Adriana Galván, "The Need for Sleep in the Adolescent Brain," *Trends in Cognitive Sciences* 24, no. 1 (January 1, 2020): 79–89, https://doi.org/10.1016/j.tics.2019.11.002

31 Shay-Ruby Wickham et al., "The Big Three Health Behaviors and Mental Health and Well-Being Among Young Adults: A Cross-Sectional Investigation of Sleep, Exercise, and Diet," *Frontiers in Psychology* 11 (2020): 579205, https://doi.org/10.3389/fpsyg.2020.579205

32 Anthony C. Rosso et al., "Frequent Restful Sleep Is Associated with the Absence of Depressive Symptoms and Higher Grade Point Average among College Students," *Sleep Health* 6, no. 5 (October 2020): 618–622, https://doi.org/10.1016/j.sleh.2020.01.018

33 Carskadon, "When Worlds Collide."

34   Mary A. Carskadon, ed., *Adolescent Sleep Patterns: Biological, Social, and Psychological Influences* (Cambridge; New York: Cambridge University Press, 2002), 19, https://doi.org/10.1017/CBO9780511499999

35   Stephanie J. Crowley et al., "An Update on Adolescent Sleep: New Evidence Informing the Perfect Storm Model," *Journal of Adolescence* 67 (August 2018): 55–65, https://doi.org/10.1016/j.adolescence.2018.06.001

36   Dement and Vaughan, *The Promise of Sleep*, 117.

37   Mary A. Carskadon, "When Worlds Collide: Adolescent Need for Sleep Versus Societal Demands," *Phi Delta Kappan* 80, no. 5 (January 1999).

38   Giovanni Farello et al., "Review of the Literature on Current Changes in the Timing of Pubertal Development and the Incomplete Forms of Early Puberty," *Frontiers in Pediatrics* 7 (2019): 147, https://doi.org/10.3389/fped.2019.00147

39   Mary A. Carskadon, Cecilia Vieira, and Christine Acebo, "Association between Puberty and Delayed Phase Preference," *Sleep* 16, no. 3 (May 1993), https://doi.org/10.1093/sleep/16.3.258.

40   Mary A. Carskadon et al., "An Approach to Studying Circadian Rhythms of Adolescent Humans," *Journal of Biological Rhythms* 12, no. 3 (June 1, 1997): 278–289, https://doi.org/10.1177/074873049701200309

41   Camilla Eckert-Lind et al., "Worldwide Secular Trends in Age at Pubertal Onset Assessed by Breast Development Among Girls: A Systematic Review and Meta-Analysis," *JAMA Pediatrics* 174, no. 4 (2020): e195881, https://doi.org/10.1001/jamapediatrics.2019.5881

42   Claes Ohlsson et al., "Secular Trends in Pubertal Growth Acceleration in Swedish Boys Born From 1947 to 1996," *JAMA Pediatrics* 173, no. 9 (2019): 860–865, https://doi.org/10.1001/jamapediatrics.2019.2315

43   Matthew D. Weaver et al., "Dose-Dependent Associations Between Sleep Duration and Unsafe Behaviors Among US High School Students," *JAMA Pediatrics* 172, no. 12 (2018): 1187–1189, https://doi.org/10.1001/jamapediatrics.2018.2777

44   Adolescent Sleep Working Group et al., "School Start Times for Adolescents," *Pediatrics* 134, no. 3 (September 2014): 642–649, https://doi.org/10.1542/peds.2014-1697

45   "Sunrise and Sunset for Minneapolis, MN," *Almanac*, August 26, 2020, https://www.almanac.com/astronomy/sun-rise-and-set/MN/Minneapolis/2020-08-26

Chapter 2: How Did We Get Here?

46   Lewis M. Terman and Adeline Hocking, "The Sleep of School Children: Its Distribution According to Age, and Its Relation to Physical and Mental Efficiency," *Journal of Educational Psychology* 4, no. 3 (1913): 138–147, https://doi.org/10.1037/h0070635

47   National Teacher and Principal Survey (NTPS), "Average Start Time and Percentage Distribution of Start Time for Public High Schools, by State: 2017–18," National Center for Education Statistics (NCES), https://nces.ed.gov/surveys/ntps/tables/ntps1718_202000602_s1s.asp

48   Thomas Hines, *The Rise and Fall of the American Teenager* (New York: Perennial, 2000), 145.

49   Ibid., 140.

50   Paula S. Fass, *The End of American Childhood: A History of Parenting from Life on the Frontier to the Managed Child* (Princeton, N.J.: Princeton University Press, 2016), 134.

51   Paul Beston, "When High Schools Shaped America's Destiny," *The Shape of Work to Come 2017*, 2017, https://www.city-journal.org/html/when-high-schools-shaped-americas-destiny-15254.html

52   Derek Thompson, "A Brief History of Teenagers," *The Saturday Evening Post*, February 13, 2018, https://www.saturdayeveningpost.com/2018/02/brief-history-teenagers/

53   Fass, *The End of American Childhood: A History of Parenting from Life on the Frontier to the Managed Child*, 128.

54   Ibid., 155.

55   Hines, *The Rise and Fall*, 252.

56   "Conant Reports Few High Schools Offer Enough Work, Special Help," *The Harvard Crimson*, January 19, 1959, https://www.thecrimson.com/article/1959/1/19/conant-reports-few-high-schools-offer/

57   William A. Fischel, "Neither 'Creatures of the State' nor 'Accidents of Geography': The Creation of American Public School Districts in the Twentieth Century," *The University of Chicago Law Review* 77, no. 1 (2010): 177–200.

58   "Transportation and School Busing: The School Bus, History of Pupil Transportation, Issues in Pupil Transportation," Education Encyclopedia—StateUniversity.com, https://education.stateuniversity.com/pages/2512/Transportation-School-Busing.html

59   Mimi Kirk, "Suburban Sprawl Stole Your Kids' Sleep," *Bloomberg CityLab*, March 23, 2017, https://www.bloomberg.com/news/articles/2017-03-23/urban-sprawl-affects-school-start-times-for-sleepy-teens

60   Judith Owens et al., "School Start Time Change: An In-Depth Examination of School Districts in the United States," *Mind, Brain, and Education* 8, no. 4 (2014): 34, https://doi.org/10.1111/mbe.12059

61   Diana Zuckerman and National Center for Health Research, "Early Morning Classes, Sleepy Students, and Risky Behaviors," *National Center for Health Research*, September 22, 2015, https://www.center4research.org/early-morning-classes-sleepy-students-risky-behaviors/

62   Jeffrey A. Groen and Sabrina Wulff Pabilonia, "Snooze or Lose: High School Start Times and Academic Achievement," *Economics of Education Review* 72 (2019): 204–218, https://doi.org/10.1016/j.econedurev.2019.05.011

63   Amy R. Wolfson and Mary A. Carskadon, "A Survey of Factors Influencing High School Start Times," *NASSP Bulletin* 89, no. 642 (March 1, 2005): 47–66, https://doi.org/10.1177/019263650508964205

64   National Teacher and Principal Survey (NTPS), "Average Start Time and Percentage Distribution of Start Time for Public High Schools, by State: 2017–18."

65 Katherine M. Keyes et al., "The Great Sleep Recession: Changes in Sleep Duration Among US Adolescents, 1991–2012," *Pediatrics* 135, no. 3 (March 2015): 460–468, https://doi.org/10.1542/peds.2014-2707

66 Jeffrey M. Jones, "In US, 40% Get Less Than Recommended Amount of Sleep," *Gallup*, December 19, 2013, https://news.gallup.com/poll/166553/less-recommended-amount-sleep.aspx

67 Tim Olds et al., "The Relationships between Sex, Age, Geography and Time in Bed in Adolescents: A Meta-Analysis of Data from 23 Countries," *Sleep Medicine Reviews* 14, no. 6 (December 2010): 371–378, https://doi.org/10.1016/j.smrv.2009.12.002

68 Kathy Sundstrom and Robert Blackmore, "Grumpy Teens, Sliding Grades? A Later Starting School Day Could Be the Answer," *ABC News*, May 6, 2019,https://www.abc.net.au/news/2019-05-07/should-high-schools-start-later/11076626

69 June C. Lo et al., "Sustained Benefits of Delaying School Start Time on Adolescent Sleep and Well-Being," *Sleep* 41, no. 6 (June 2018), https://doi.org/10.1093/sleep/zsy052

70 National Teacher and Principal Survey (NTPS), "Average Start Time and Percentage Distribution of Start Time for Public High Schools, by State: 2017–18."

71 Geneviève Gariépy et al., "School Start Time and Sleep in Canadian Adolescents," *Journal of Sleep Research* 26, no. 2 (November 23, 2016): 195–201, https://doi.org/10.1111/jsr.12475

72 Geneviève Gariépy et al., "How Are Adolescents Sleeping? Adolescent Sleep Patterns and Sociodemographic Differences in 24 European and North American Countries," *Journal of Adolescent Health* 66, no. 6 (June 1, 2020): S81–88, https://doi.org/10.1016/j.jadohealth.2020.03.013

Chapter 3: Taking It to the Schools

73 Duchesne P. Drew, "High School Start Times under Review," *Star Tribune*, December 10, 1996.

74 Kyla Wahlstrom, "Changing Times: Findings from the First Longitudinal Study of Later High School Start Times," *NASSP Bulletin* 86, no. 633 (December 1, 2002): 16, https://doi.org/10.1177/019263650208663302

75 Zoe Lofgren, "H.R.1861—ZZZ's to A's Act—116th Congress (2019-2020)" (2019), https://www.congress.gov/bill/116th-congress/house-bill/1861/text

76 Dara O'Brien, "Taking Sleep Public," *Sleep Review*, August 28, 2014, https://sleepreviewmag.com/sleep-health/sleep-whole-body/taking-sleep-public-cdc-wayne-giles/

77 Kyla Wahlstrom et al., "Examining the Impact of Later High School Start Times on the Health and Academic Performance of High School Students: A Multi-Site Study," report (St. Paul, MN: Center for Applied Research and Educational Improvement. University of Minnesota, February 2014), https://hdl.handle.net/11299/162769

78 Judith Owens et al., "School Start Time Change: An In-Depth Examination of School Districts in the United States," *Mind, Brain, and Education* 8, no. 4 (2014), https://doi.org/10.1111/mbe.12059

79   Adolescent Sleep Working Group et al., "School Start Times for Adolescents," *Pediatrics* 134, no. 3 (September 2014): 642–649, https://doi.org/10.1542/peds.2014-1697

80   CDC Newsroom, "Students Need Adequate Sleep for Their Health, Safety, and Academic Success (Press Release)," Centers for Disease Control and Prevention (CDC), August 6, 2015, https://www.cdc.gov/media/releases/2015/p0806-school-sleep.html

Chapter 4: Sleep and Mental Health

81   Taylor Chiu, "Taylor Parker Chiu—Out of the Darkness," *Momentum for Health*, September 25, 2015, https://momentumforhealth.org/taylor-chiu-out-of-the-darkness

82   MMWR and Centers for Disease Control and Prevention (CDC), "Reports, Fact Sheets, and Publications | YRBSS | Adolescent and School Health | CDC."

83   Jay Giedd, "The Amazing Teen Brain," *Scientific American* 312, no. 6 (May 19, 2015): 32–37, https://doi.org/10.1038/scientificamerican0615-32

84   Laurence D. Steinberg, *Age of Opportunity: Lessons from the New Science of Adolescence* (Boston: Houghton Mifflin Harcourt, 2015), 71.

85   Z. Krizan, A. Miller, and G. Hisler, "Does Losing Sleep Unleash Anger?," *Sleep* 43, no. S1 (April 2020): A105, https://doi.org/10.1093/sleep/zsaa056.274

86   Osamu Itani et al., "Anger and Impulsivity Among Japanese Adolescents: A Nationwide Representative Survey," *The Journal of Clinical Psychiatry* 77, no. 7 (July 27, 2016): e860-866, https://doi.org/10.4088/JCP.15m10044

87   S. V. Bauducco et al., "Sleep Duration and Patterns in Adolescents: Correlates and the Role of Daily Stressors," *Sleep Health* 2, no. 3 (September 1, 2016): 211–218, https://doi.org/10.1016/j.sleh.2016.05.006

88   Michelle A. Short et al., "The Relationship Between Sleep Duration and Mood in Adolescents: A Systematic Review and Meta-Analysis," *Sleep Medicine Reviews* 52 (August 1, 2020): 101311, https://doi.org/10.1016/j.smrv.2020.101311

89   Faith Orchard et al., "Self-Reported Sleep Patterns and Quality Amongst Adolescents: Cross-Sectional and Prospective Associations with Anxiety and Depression," *Journal of Child Psychology and Psychiatry* 61, no. 10 (2020): 1126-1137, https://doi.org/10.1111/jcpp.13288

90   CDC Injury Prevention & Control, "Web-Based Injury Statistics Query and Reporting System (WISQARS)—Data and Statistics," *Centers for Disease Control and Prevention*, https://www.cdc.gov/injury/wisqars/index.html

91   Adam Winsler et al., "Sleepless in Fairfax: The Difference One More Hour of Sleep Can Make for Teen Hopelessness, Suicidal Ideation, and Substance Use," *Journal of Youth and Adolescence* 44, no. 2 (February 1, 2015): 362–378, https://doi.org/10.1007/s10964-014-0170-3

92   Matthew D. Weaver et al., "Dose-Dependent Associations Between Sleep Duration and Unsafe Behaviors Among US High School Students," *JAMA Pediatrics* 172, no. 12 (2018): 1187–1189, https://doi.org/10.1001/jamapediatrics.2018.2777

93   MMWR and Centers for Disease Control and Prevention (CDC), "Reports, Fact Sheets, and Publications | YRBSS | Adolescent and School Health | CDC."

94 Hsiao-Yean Chiu et al., "Associations between Sleep Duration and Suicidality in Adolescents: A Systematic Review and Dose-Response Meta-Analysis," *Sleep Medicine Reviews* 42 (December 2018): 119–126, https://doi.org/10.1016/j. smrv.2018.07.003

95 Matthew P. Walker, *Why We Sleep: Unlocking the Power of Sleep and Dreams* (New York, NY: Scribner, an imprint of Simon & Schuster, Inc., 2017), 215-216.

96 N. L. Sin et al., "Day-to-Day Associations between Sleep Quality and Daily Experiences in Youth" (Paper session at the SLEEP Meeting of the Associated Professional Sleep Societies, Seattle, WA., 2015).

97 Yijie Wang and Tiffany Yip, "Sleep Facilitates Coping: Moderated Mediation of Daily Sleep, Ethnic/Racial Discrimination, Stress Responses, and Adolescent Well-Being," *Child Development* 91, no. 4 (2020): e833–852, https://doi.org/10.1111/cdev.13324

98 Amanda E. Chue et al., "The Role of Sleep in Adolescents' Daily Stress Recovery: Negative Affect Spillover and Positive Affect Bounce-Back Effects," *Journal of Adolescence* 66 (July 2018): 101–111, https://doi.org/10.1016/j. adolescence.2018.05.006

99 Shay-Ruby Wickham et al., "The Big Three Health Behaviors and Mental Health and Well-Being Among Young Adults: A Cross-Sectional Investigation of Sleep, Exercise, and Diet," *Frontiers in Psychology* 11 (2020): 579205, https://doi.org/10.3389/ fpsyg.2020.579205

Chapter 5: Risky Behaviors and Unhealthy Habits

100 Abigail A. Baird, Jonathan A. Fugelsang, and Craig M. Bennett, " 'What Were You Thinking'?: An FMRI Study of Adolescent Decision Making" (Hannover, NH.: Department of Psychological and Brain Sciences, Dartmouth College, January 2005).

101 Laurence D. Steinberg, *Age of Opportunity: Lessons from the New Science of Adolescence* (Boston: Houghton Mifflin Harcourt, 2015), 73.

102 Laurence Steinberg et al., "Around the World, Adolescence Is a Time of Heightened Sensation Seeking and Immature Self-Regulation," *Developmental Science* 21, no. 2 (2018): e12532, https://doi.org/10.1111/desc.12532

103 Jennifer L. Robinson et al., "Neurophysiological Differences in the Adolescent Brain Following a Single Night of Restricted Sleep—A 7T fMRI Study," *Developmental Cognitive Neuroscience* 31, no. C (April 1, 2018), https://doi.org/10.1016/j. dcn.2018.03.012

104 Adriana Galván, "The Unrested Adolescent Brain," *Child Development Perspectives* 13, no. 3 (June 25, 2019): 141–146, https://doi.org/10.1111/cdep.12332

105 Ryan C. Meldrum, J. C. Barnes, and Carter Hay, "Sleep Deprivation, Low Self-Control, and Delinquency: A Test of the Strength Model of Self-Control," *Journal of Youth and Adolescence* 44, no. 2 (February 1, 2015): 465–477, https://doi. org/10.1007/s10964-013-0024-4

106 Daniel C. Semenza et al., "Adolescent Sleep Problems and Susceptibility to Peer Influence," *Youth & Society*, (November 2, 2020), https://doi. org/10.1177/0044118X20969024

107 Daniel C. Semenza et al., "School Start Times, Delinquency, and Substance Use: A Criminological Perspective," *Crime & Delinquency* 66, no. 2 (February 1, 2020): 163–193, https://doi.org/10.1177/0011128719845147

108 Office of Juvenile Justice and Delinquency Prevention (OJJDP), "Statistical Briefing Book: Juvenile Violent Crime Time of Day," *Office of Justice Programs. US Department of Justice*, https://www.ojjdp.gov/ojstatbb/offenders/qa03301.asp?qaDate=2016

109 Ryan Charles Meldrum and Emily Restivo, "The Behavioral and Health Consequences of Sleep Deprivation Among US High School Students: Relative Deprivation Matters," *Preventive Medicine* 63 (June 2014): 24–28, https://doi.org/10.1016/j.ypmed.2014.03.006

110 Wendy M. Troxel, Brett Ewing, and Elizabeth J. D'Amico, "Examining Racial/Ethnic Disparities in the Association between Adolescent Sleep and Alcohol or Marijuana Use," *Sleep Health* 1, no. 2 (June 2015): 104–108, https://doi.org/10.1016/j.sleh.2015.03.005

111 Matthew D. Weaver et al., "Dose-Dependent Associations Between Sleep Duration and Unsafe Behaviors Among US High School Students," *JAMA Pediatrics* 172, no. 12 (2018): 1187–1189, https://doi.org/10.1001/jamapediatrics.2018.2777

112 Ibid.

113 Frances E. Jensen and Amy Ellis Nutt, *The Teenage Brain: A Neuroscientist's Survival Guide to Raising Adolescents and Young Adults* (New York, NY: Harper, 2015), 165.

114 Carolin F. Reichert et al., "Wide Awake at Bedtime? Effects of Caffeine on Sleep and Circadian Timing in Male Adolescents – A Randomized Crossover Trial," *Biochemical Pharmacology* 191 (September 2021): 114283, https://doi.org/10.1016/j.bcp.2020.114283

115 Kathleen E. Miller, Kurt H. Dermen, and Joseph F. Lucke, "Caffeinated Energy Drink Use by US Adolescents Aged 13–17: A National Profile," *Psychology of Addictive Behaviors* 32, no. 6 (September 2018): 647–659, https://doi.org/10.1037/adb0000389

116 Cecile A. Marczinski, "Alcohol Mixed with Energy Drinks: Consumption Patterns and Motivations for Use in US College Students," *International Journal of Environmental Research and Public Health* 8, no. 8 (August 2011): 3232–3245, https://doi.org/10.3390/ijerph8083232

117 Bingqian Zhu et al., "Effects of Sleep Restriction on Metabolism-Related Parameters in Healthy Adults: A Comprehensive Review and Meta-Analysis of Randomized Controlled Trials," *Sleep Medicine Reviews* 45 (June 2019): 18–30, https://doi.org/10.1016/j.smrv.2019.02.002

118 Jean-Philippe Chaput and Caroline Dutil, "Lack of Sleep as a Contributor to Obesity in Adolescents: Impacts on Eating and Activity Behaviors," *International Journal of Behavioral Nutrition and Physical Activity* 13, no. 1 (September 26, 2016): 103, https://doi.org/10.1186/s12966-016-0428-0

119 Eri Tajiri et al., "Acute Sleep Curtailment Increases Sweet Taste Preference, Appetite and Food Intake in Healthy Young Adults: A Randomized Crossover Trial," *Behavioral Sciences* 10, no. 2 (February 2020): 47, https://doi.org/10.3390/bs10020047

120 Stacey L. Simon et al., "Sweet/Dessert Foods Are More Appealing to Adolescents after Sleep Restriction," *PLOS ONE* 10, no. 2 (February 23, 2015): e0115434, https://doi.org/10.1371/journal.pone.0115434

121 Rachel Widome et al., "Sleep Duration and Weight-Related Behaviors among Adolescents," *Childhood Obesity* 15, no. 7 (October 2019): 434–442, https://doi.org/10.1089/chi.2018.0362

122 Matthew P. Walker, *Why We Sleep: Unlocking the Power of Sleep and Dreams* (New York, NY: Scribner, an imprint of Simon & Schuster, Inc., 2017), 177.

123 Tracey J. Smith et al., "Impact of Sleep Restriction on Local Immune Response and Skin Barrier Restoration With and Without 'Multinutrient' Nutrition Intervention," *Journal of Applied Physiology* 124, no. 1 (January 2018): 190–200, https://doi.org/10.1152/japplphysiol.00547.2017

124 Lisa Marie Potter and Nicholas Weiler, "Short Sleepers Are Four Times More Likely to Catch a Cold," *UC San Francisco*, August 31, 2015, https://www.ucsf.edu/news/2015/08/131411/short-sleepers-are-four-times-more-likely-catch-cold

125 Aric A. Prather et al., "Temporal Links Between Self-Reported Sleep and Antibody Responses to the Influenza Vaccine," *International Journal of Behavioral Medicine* 28, no. 1 (February 2021): 151–158, https://doi.org/10.1007/s12529-020-09879-4

126 Brandon R. Reynolds, "New Study Will Examine How Robustly Individuals Respond to COVID-19 Vaccination," *UC San Francisco*, March 3, 2021, https://www.ucsf.edu/news/2021/03/419971/new-study-will-examine-how-robustly-individuals-respond-covid-19-vaccination

Chapter 6: Sleepwalking through School

127 Mary A. Carskadon, ed., *Adolescent Sleep Patterns: Biological, Social, and Psychological Influences* (Cambridge; New York: Cambridge University Press, 2002), 127, https://doi.org/10.1017/CBO9780511499999

128 Gideon P. Dunster et al., "Sleepmore in Seattle: Later School Start Times Are Associated with More Sleep and Better Performance in High School Students," *Science Advances* 4, no. 12 (December 1, 2018): eaau6200, https://doi.org/10.1126/sciadv.aau6200

129 Brian A. Jacob and Jonah E. Rockoff, "Organizing Schools to Improve Student Achievement: Start Times, Grade Configurations, and Teacher Assignments," *Brookings* (blog), September 27, 2011, https://www.brookings.edu/research/organizing-schools-to-improve-student-achievement-start-times-grade-configurations-and-teacher-assignments/

130 Lauren Hale and Wendy Troxel, "Embracing the School Start Later Movement: Adolescent Sleep Deprivation as a Public Health and Social Justice Problem," *American Journal of Public Health* 108, no. 5 (May 2018): 599–600, https://doi.org/10.2105/AJPH.2018.304381

131 Kyla Wahlstrom, "Changing Times: Findings from the First Longitudinal Study of Later High School Start Times," *NASSP Bulletin* 86, no. 633 (December 1, 2002), https://doi.org/10.1177/019263650208663302

132 Pamela V. Thacher and Serge V. Onyper, "Longitudinal Outcomes of Start Time Delay on Sleep, Behavior, and Achievement in High School," *Sleep* 39, no. 2 (February 2016): 271–281, https://doi.org/10.5665/sleep.5426

133 Pamela Malaspina McKeever and Linda Clark, "Delayed High School Start Times Later than 8:30 a.m. and Impact on Graduation Rates and Attendance Rates," *Sleep Health* 3, no. 2 (April 1, 2017): 119–125, https://doi.org/10.1016/j.sleh.2017.01.002

134 Mary A. Carskadon, "Sleep's Effects on Cognition and Learning in Adolescence," in *Human Sleep and Cognition Part II: Clinical and Applied Research*, ed. Hans P. A. Van Dongen and Gerard A. Kerkhof, *Progress in Brain Research 190* (Amsterdam; London: Elsevier Science, 2011), 137–143.

135 Kyla Wahlstrom et al., "Examining the Impact of Later High School Start Times on the Health and Academic Performance of High School Students: A Multi-Site Study," report (St. Paul, MN: Center for Applied Research and Educational Improvement. University of Minnesota, February 2014), https://hdl.handle.net/11299/162769

136 Kyla L. Wahlstrom, "Later Start Time for Teens Improves Grades, Mood, and Safety," *Phi Delta Kappan* 98, no. 4 (December 1, 2016): 8–14.

137 Guifeng Xu et al., "Twenty-Year Trends in Diagnosed Attention-Deficit/Hyperactivity Disorder Among US Children and Adolescents, 1997-2016," *JAMA Network Open* 1, no. 4 (August 31, 2018): 1997–2016, https://doi.org/10.1001/jamanetworkopen.2018.1471

138 Hawley Montgomery-Downs, ed., *Sleep Science* (New York, NY: Oxford University Press, 2020), 344.

139 Reut Gruber et al., "Short Sleep Duration Is Associated with Teacher-Reported Inattention and Cognitive Problems in Healthy School-Aged Children," *Nature and Science of Sleep* 4 (March 7, 2012): 33–40, https://doi.org/10.2147/NSS.S24607

140 Jenny Dimakos et al., "The Associations Between Sleep and Externalizing and Internalizing Problems in Children and Adolescents with Attention-Deficit/Hyperactivity Disorder: Empirical Findings, Clinical Implications, and Future Research Directions," *Child and Adolescent Psychiatric Clinics of North America*, Sleep Disorders in Children and Adolescents, 30, no. 1 (January 2021): 175–193, https://doi.org/10.1016/j.chc.2020.08.001

141 McKeever and Clark, "Delayed High School Start Times Later than 8."

142 Teny M. Shapiro, "The Educational Effects of School Start Times," *IZA World of Labor*, no. 181 (August 1, 2015), https://doi.org/10.15185/izawol.181

143 Marco Hafner, Martin Stepanek, and Wendy M. Troxel, "Later School Start Times in the US: An Economic Analysis" (RAND Corporation, August 30, 2017).

144 Andrew J. Fuligni et al., "Adolescent Sleep Duration, Variability, and Peak Levels of Achievement and Mental Health," *Child Development* 89, no. 2 (2018): e18–28, https://doi.org/10.1111/cdev.12729.

145 Douglas Martin, "Late to Bed, Early to Rise Makes a Teen-Ager...Tired," *The New York Times*, August 1, 1999, https://www.nytimes.com/1999/08/01/education/late-to-bed-early-to-rise-makes-a-teen-ager-tired.html

Chapter 7: Sleep and Sports

146 Cheri D. Mah et al., "The Effects of Sleep Extension on the Athletic Performance of Collegiate Basketball Players," *Sleep* 34, no. 7 (July 2011): 943–950, https://doi.org/10.5665/SLEEP.1132

147 Jason J. Jones et al., "Association between Late-Night Tweeting and Next-Day Game Performance Among Professional Basketball Players," *Sleep Health* 5, no. 1 (February 2019): 68–71, https://doi.org/10.1016/j.sleh.2018.09.005

148 American Academy of Sleep Medicine, "Fatigue and Sleep Linked to Major League Baseball Performance and Career Longevity," *ScienceDaily*, May 31, 2013, https://www.sciencedaily.com/releases/2013/05/130531105506.htm

149 Matthew D. Milewski et al., "Chronic Lack of Sleep Is Associated with Increased Sports Injuries in Adolescent Athletes," *Journal of Pediatric Orthopedics* 34, no. 2 (March 2014): 129–133, https://doi.org/10.1097/BPO.0000000000000151

150 Zachary Y. Kerr et al., "Concussion Incidence and Trends in 20 High School Sports," *Pediatrics* 144, no. 5 (November 1, 2019): e20192180, https://doi.org/10.1542/peds.2019-2180

151 Adam C. Raikes et al., "Insomnia and Daytime Sleepiness: Risk Factors for Sports-Related Concussion," *Sleep Medicine* 58 (June 2019): 66–74, https://doi.org/10.1016/j.sleep.2019.03.008

152 Ibid.

Chapter 8: Teens and Drowsy Driving

153 Samantha Tatro, " 'I Shouldn't Be Here': Teen, Asleep at Wheel, Nearly Impaled by Fence," *NBC 7 (San Diego)*, June 2, 2015, https://www.nbcsandiego.com/news/local/i-shouldnt-be-here-teen-asleep-at-wheel-nearly-impaled-by-fence/98261/

154 National Highway Traffic Safety Administration (NHTSA), "Asleep at The Wheel: A National Compendium of Efforts to Eliminate Drowsy Driving" (US Department of Transportation, March 2017), 24.

155 Justin M. Owens et al., "Prevalence of Drowsy Driving Crashes: Estimates from a Large-Scale Naturalistic Driving Study (Research Brief)" (Washington, DC: AAA Foundation for Traffic Safety, February 8, 2018), https://aaafoundation.org/prevalence-drowsy-driving-crashes-estimates-large-scale-naturalistic-driving-study/

156 Brian C. Tefft, "Acute Sleep Deprivation and Culpable Motor Vehicle Crash Involvement," *Sleep* 41, no. 10 (October 1, 2018): zsy144, https://doi.org/10.1093/sleep/zsy144

157 AAA Foundation for Traffic Safety, "2019 Traffic Safety Culture Index" (Washington, DC: AAA Foundation for Traffic Safety, June 2020), https://newsroom.aaa.com/wp-content/uploads/2020/10/2019-TSCI-Report-_AAAFTS-0601.pdf

158 CDC Transportation Safety, "Teen Drivers: Get the Facts," *Centers for Disease Control and Prevention*, October 12, 2021, https://www.cdc.gov/transportationsafety/teen_drivers/teendrivers_factsheet.html

159 National Center for Health Statistics (NCHS), "10 Leading Causes of Injury Deaths by Age Group Highlighting Unintentional Injury Deaths, United States—2018," *Centers for Disease Control and Prevention*, 2018, https://www.cdc.gov/injury/images/lc-charts/leading_causes_of_death_by_age_group_unintentional_2018_1100w850h.jpg

160 National Center for Statistics and Analysis, "Young Drivers: 2018 Data. (Traffic Safety Facts, Report No. DO HS 812 968)" (National Highway Traffic Safety Administration, October 2020), https://crashstats.nhtsa.dot.gov/Api/Public/ViewPublication/812968

161 Andrew Gross, "A Perfect Storm? COVID-19 Restrictions Ease As '100 Deadliest Days' Begin for Nation's Teens," *AAA Newsroom*, May 27, 2020, https://newsroom.aaa. com/2020/05/a-perfect-storm-covid-19-restrictions-ease-as-100-deadliest-days-begin-for-nations-teens/

162 CDC Transportation Safety, "Teen Drivers."

163 Insurance Institute for Highway Safety (IIHS) and Highway Loss Data Institute (HLDI), "Teenagers: Graduated Licensing Laws by State," *IIHS-HLDI*, December 2021, https://www.iihs.org/topics/teenagers/graduated-licensing-laws-table

164 Jonathan Fu et al., "The Impact of State Level Graduated Driver Licensing Programs on Rates of Passenger Restraint Use and Unlicensed Driving in Fatal Crashes," *Annals of Advances in Automotive Medicine* 57 (September 2013): 89–98.

165 David S. Hurwitz et al., "Improving Teenage Driver Perceptions Regarding the Impact of Distracted Driving in the Pacific Northwest," *Journal of Transportation Safety & Security* 8, no. 2 (April 2, 2016): 148–163, https://doi.org/10.1080/19439962 .2014.997329

166 Matthew D. Weaver et al., "Dose-Dependent Associations Between Sleep Duration and Unsafe Behaviors Among US High School Students," *JAMA Pediatrics* 172, no. 12 (2018): 1187–1189, https://doi.org/10.1001/jamapediatrics.2018.2777

167 Michael Dreyfuss et al., "Teens Impulsively React Rather than Retreat from Threat," *Developmental Neuroscience* 36, no. 3–4 (2014): 220–227, https://doi. org/10.1159/000357755

168 Z. Krizan, A. Miller, and G. Hisler, "Does Losing Sleep Unleash Anger?," *Sleep* 43, no. S1 (April 2020): A105, https://doi.org/10.1093/sleep/zsaa056.274

169 Michelle A. Short et al., "Estimating Adolescent Sleep Need Using Dose-Response Modeling," *Sleep* 41, no. 4 (April 1, 2018): zsy011, https://doi.org/10.1093/ sleep/zsy011

170 Robert D. Foss, Richard L. Smith, and Natalie P. O'Brien, "School Start Times and Teenage Driver Motor Vehicle Crashes," *Accident Analysis & Prevention* 126 (May 1, 2019): 54–63, https://doi.org/10.1016/j.aap.2018.03.031

171 Kyla Wahlstrom et al., "Examining the Impact of Later High School Start Times on the Health and Academic Performance of High School Students: A Multi-Site Study," report (St. Paul, MN: Center for Applied Research and Educational Improvement. University of Minnesota, February 2014), https://hdl.handle.net/11299/162769

172 Robert Daniel Vorona et al., "Adolescent Crash Rates and School Start Times in Two Central Virginia Counties, 2009-2011: A Follow-up Study to a Southeastern Virginia Study, 2007-2008," *Journal of Clinical Sleep Medicine* 10, no. 11 (November 15, 2014): 1169–1177, https://doi.org/10.5664/jcsm.4192

173 Alexandra L. C. Martiniuk et al., "Sleep-Deprived Young Drivers and the Risk for Crash: The DRIVE Prospective Cohort Study," *JAMA Pediatrics* 167, no. 7 (July 2013): 647–655, https://doi.org/10.1001/jamapediatrics.2013.1429

Chapter 9: Not All Teens Sleep the Same

174 Massimiliano de Zambotti et al., "The Falling Asleep Process in Adolescents," *Sleep* 43, no. 6 (June 15, 2020): zsz312, https://doi.org/10.1093/sleep/zsz312

175 Dilara Yuksel et al., "Stress, Sleep, and Autonomic Function in Healthy Adolescent Girls and Boys: Findings from the NCANDA Study," *Sleep Health* 7, no. 1 (Feb. 1, 2021): https://doi.org/10.1016/j.sleh.2020.06.004

176 Vincenzo De Sanctis et al., "Primary Dysmenorrhea in Adolescents: Prevalence, Impact and Recent Knowledge," *Pediatric Endocrinology Reviews* 13, no. 2 (December 2015): 512–520.

177 Xianchen Liu et al., "Early Menarche and Menstrual Problems Are Associated with Sleep Disturbance in a Large Sample of Chinese Adolescent Girls," *Sleep* 40, no. 9 (September 1, 2017): zsx107, https://doi.org/10.1093/sleep/zsx107

178 Gladys M. Martinez, "Trends and Patterns in Menarche in the United States: 1995 through 2013-2017," *National Health Statistics Reports*, no. 146 (September 2020): 1–12.

179 Ga Eun Nam, Kyungdo Han, and Gyungjoo Lee, "Association Between Sleep Duration and Menstrual Cycle Irregularity in Korean Female Adolescents," *Sleep Medicine* 35 (July 2017): 62–66, https://doi.org/10.1016/j.sleep.2017.04.009

180 Yoko Komada et al., "Social Jetlag and Menstrual Symptoms Among Female University Students," *Chronobiology International* 36, no. 2 (February 2019): 258–264, https://doi.org/10.1080/07420528.2018.1533561

181 Devorah Heitner, "Is Instagram Bad for Kids? What Parents Can Do," *Raising Digital Natives*, October 1, 2021, https://www.raisingdigitalnatives.com/instagram-and-kids/

182 Sharon Goulds et al., *Free to Be Online? Girls' and Young Women's Experiences of Online Harassment* (Plan International; Girls get Equal, 2020), https://plan-international.org/publications/freetobeonline

183 Liisa Kuula, Timo Partonen, and Anu-Katriina Pesonen, "Emotions Relating to Romantic Love—Further Disruptors of Adolescent Sleep," *Sleep Health* 6, no. 2 (April 1, 2020): 159–165, https://doi.org/10.1016/j.sleh.2020.01.006

184 Jeffrey M. Jones, "LGBT Identification Rises to 5.6% in Latest US Estimate," *Gallup*, February 24, 2021, https://news.gallup.com/poll/329708/lgbt-identification-rises-latest-estimate.aspx

185 MMWR and Centers for Disease Control and Prevention (CDC), "Reports, Fact Sheets, and Publications | YRBSS | Adolescent and School Health | CDC."

186 Human Rights Campaign (HRC), "2018 LGBTQ Youth Report" (Human Rights Campaign, 2018), https://www.hrc.org/resources/2018-lgbtq-youth-report

187 Pengsheng Li et al., "Is Sexual Minority Status Associated with Poor Sleep Quality Among Adolescents? Analysis of a National Cross-Sectional Survey in Chinese Adolescents," *BMJ Open* 7, no. 12 (December 1, 2017): e017067, https://doi.org/10.1136/bmjopen-2017-017067

188 Eliana S. Butler, Eleanor McGlinchey, and Robert-Paul Juster, "Sexual and Gender Minority Sleep: A Narrative Review and Suggestions for Future Research," *Journal of Sleep Research* 29, no. 1 (2020): e12928, https://doi.org/10.1111/jsr.12928

189 Emma Potter and Charlotte Patterson, "Sexual Orientation and Short Sleep Among Adults: Differences Across and Within Racial/Ethnic Groups," in *APHA's 2019 Annual Meeting and Expo*, 2019, https://apha.confex.com/apha/2019/meetingapi.cgi/Paper/445658?filename=2019_Abstract445658.html&template=Word

190 MMWR and Centers for Disease Control and Prevention (CDC), "Reports, Fact Sheets, and Publications | YRBSS | Adolescent and School Health | CDC."

191 Brian Resnick, "The Racial Inequality of Sleep," *The Atlantic*, October 27, 2015, https://www.theatlantic.com/health/archive/2015/10/the-sleep-gap-and-racial-inequality/412405/

192 Dana Guglielmo et al., "Racial/Ethnic Sleep Disparities in US School-Aged Children and Adolescents: A Review of the Literature," *Sleep Health* 4, no. 1 (February 2018): 68–80, https://doi.org/10.1016/j.sleh.2017.09.005

193 Tiffany Yip et al., "Racial Disparities in Sleep: Associations with Discrimination Among Ethnic/Racial Minority Adolescents," *Child Development* 91, no. 3 (2020): 914–931, https://doi.org/10.1111/cdev.13234

194 J. Michael Underwood et al., "Overview and Methods for the Youth Risk Behavior Surveillance System—United States, 2019," *MMWR Supplements* 69, no. 1 (2020): 1–10, https://doi.org/10.15585/mmwr.su6901a1

195 Tiffany Yip et al., "Sociodemographic and Environmental Factors Associated with Childhood Sleep Duration," *Sleep Health* 6, no. 6 (December 2020): 767–777, https://doi.org/10.1016/j.sleh.2020.05.007

196 Yip et al., "Racial Disparities in Sleep."

197 Tiffany Yip et al., "Discrimination and Sleep Mediate Ethnic/Racial Identity and Adolescent Adjustment: Uncovering Change Processes with Slope-as-Mediator Mediation," *Child Development* 91, no. 3 (2020): 1021–1043, https://doi.org/10.1111/cdev.13276

198 Philip Cheng et al., "Racial Discrimination as a Mediator of Racial Disparities in Insomnia Disorder," *Sleep Health* 6, no. 5 (October 1, 2020): 543–549, https://doi.org/10.1016/j.sleh.2020.07.007

199 Lianne Tomfohr et al., "Racial Differences in Sleep Architecture: The Role of Ethnic Discrimination," *Biological Psychology* 89, no. 1 (January 1, 2012): 34–38, https://doi.org/10.1016/j.biopsycho.2011.09.002

200 Kiara Wyndham Douds and Michael Hout, "Microaggressions in the United States," *Sociological Science* 7 (November 2, 2020): 528–543, https://doi.org/10.15195/v7.a22

201 Aprile D. Benner et al., "Racial/Ethnic Discrimination and Well-Being during Adolescence: A Meta-Analytic Review," *American Psychologist* 73, no. 7 (October 2018): 855–883, https://doi.org/10.1037/amp0000204

202 Maximus Berger and Zoltán Sarnyai, " 'More than Skin Deep': Stress Neurobiology and Mental Health Consequences of Racial Discrimination," *Stress* 18, no. 1 (January 2015): 1–10, https://doi.org/10.3109/10253890.2014.989204

203 "Ethnic and Racial Minorities & Socioeconomic Status," *American Psychological Association*, July 2017, https://www.apa.org/pi/ses/resources/publications/minorities

204 Megan E. Petrov et al., "Racial Differences in Sleep Duration Intersect with Sex, Socioeconomic Status, and US Geographic Region: The REGARDS Study," *Sleep Health* 6, no. 4 (August 1, 2020): 442–450, https://doi.org/10.1016/j.sleh.2020.05.004

205 Michael A. Grandner et al., "Sleep Symptoms, Race/Ethnicity, and Socioeconomic Position," *Journal of Clinical Sleep Medicine* 09, no. 09 (September 15, 2013): 897–905, https://doi.org/10.5664/jcsm.2990

206 Alisha Coleman-Jensen et al., "Household Food Security in the United States in 2019," Economic Research Report (US Department of Agriculture, September 2020), http://www.ers.usda.gov/publications/pub-details/?pubid=99281

207 Alisha Coleman-Jensen et al., "Household Food Security in the United States in 2020," Economic Research Report (US Department of Agriculture, September 2021), https://www.ers.usda.gov/publications/pub-details/?pubid=102075

208 Jason M. Nagata et al., "Food Insecurity Is Associated with Poorer Mental Health and Sleep Outcomes in Young Adults," *Journal of Adolescent Health* 65, no. 6 (December 1, 2019): 805–811, https://doi.org/10.1016/j.jadohealth.2019.08.010

209 Dietary Guidelines for Americans (DGA), "Home | Dietary Guidelines for Americans (2020-2025)," *Dietary Guidelines for Americans*, 2020, https://www.dietaryguidelines.gov/

210 Robert Bozick, Wendy M. Troxel, and Lynn A. Karoly, "Housing Insecurity and Sleep among Welfare Recipients in California," *Sleep* 44, no. 7 (July 1, 2021): zsab005, https://doi.org/10.1093/sleep/zsab005

211 Brian Resnick and *National Journal*, "The Black-White Sleep Gap," *The Atlantic*, October 23, 2015, https://www.theatlantic.com/politics/archive/2015/10/the-black-white-sleep-gap/454311/

212 Nakayla Griffin et al., "Aspects of Disordered Neighborhoods Are Associated with Insomnia, Sleepiness, Fatigue and Control Over Sleep," *Sleep* 42, no. S1 (April 12, 2019): A86, https://doi.org/10.1093/sleep/zsz067.208

213 Ryan Charles Meldrum et al., "Perceived School Safety, Perceived Neighborhood Safety, and Insufficient Sleep among Adolescents," *Sleep Health* 4, no. 5 (October 2018): 429–435, https://doi.org/10.1016/j.sleh.2018.07.006

214 Connor Sheehan et al., "Historical Neighborhood Poverty Trajectories and Child Sleep," *Sleep Health* 4, no. 2 (April 2018): 127–134, https://doi.org/10.1016/j.sleh.2017.12.005

Chapter 10: How to Help Teens Get More Sleep: Daytime Considerations

215 Stacy B. Dale and Alan B. Krueger, "Estimating the Effects of College Characteristics Over the Career Using Administrative Earnings Data," *The Journal of Human Resources* 49, no. 2 (2014): 323–358.

216 Challenge Success, "Quality Over Quantity: Elements of Effective Homework" (Stanford University Graduate School of Education, August 2020), https://challengesuccess.org/wp-content/uploads/2021/04/Challenge-Success-Homework-White-Paper-2020.pdf

217 Sing Chen Yeo et al., "Associations of Time Spent on Homework or Studying with Nocturnal Sleep Behavior and Depression Symptoms in Adolescents from Singapore," *Sleep Health* 6, no. 6 (December 1, 2020): 758–766, https://doi.org/10.1016/j.sleh.2020.04.011

218 Dave Philipps, "The Army Rolls Out a New Weapon: Strategic Napping," *The New York Times*, October 1, 2020, https://www.nytimes.com/2020/10/01/us/army-naps.html

219 June C. Lo et al., "Neurobehavioral Impact of Successive Cycles of Sleep Restriction With and Without Naps in Adolescents," *Sleep* 40, no. 2 (February 1, 2017): zsw042, https://doi.org/10.1093/sleep/zsw042

220 Matthew P. Walker, *Why We Sleep: Unlocking the Power of Sleep and Dreams* (New York, NY: Scribner, an imprint of Simon & Schuster, Inc., 2017), 28.

221 "Take a Caffeine Nap (Really!)," *Railroaders' Guide to Healthy Sleep*, https://railroadersleep.fra.dot.gov/Improve/Smart-Sleep-Tips-A-to-Zzzzz/Use-Caffeine-Wisely/Take-a-Caffeine-Nap-Really

222 Joseph Stromberg, "Scientists Agree: Coffee Naps Are Better than Coffee or Naps Alone," *Vox*, April 23, 2015, https://www.vox.com/2014/8/28/6074177/coffee-naps-caffeine-science

223 Lindsay Master et al., "Bidirectional, Daily Temporal Associations between Sleep and Physical Activity in Adolescents," *Scientific Reports* 9, no. 1 (May 22, 2019): 7732, https://doi.org/10.1038/s41598-019-44059-9

224 Rafael Pelayo, *How to Sleep: The New Science-Based Solutions for Sleeping Through the Night* (New York, NY: Artisan Books, a division of Workman Publishing Co., 2020), 58.

225 Caitlin L. Merlo et al., "Dietary and Physical Activity Behaviors Among High School Students—Youth Risk Behavior Survey, United States, 2019," *MMWR Supplements* 69, no. 1 (August 21, 2020): 64–76, https://doi.org/10.15585/mmwr.su6901a8

Chapter 11: Other Ways to Help Teens Get More Sleep: Night Moves

226 Matthew P. Walker, *Why We Sleep: Unlocking the Power of Sleep and Dreams* (New York, NY: Scribner, an imprint of Simon & Schuster, Inc., 2017), 112.

227 Sha Huang et al., "Sleep Restriction Impairs Vocabulary Learning When Adolescents Cram for Exams: The Need for Sleep Study," *Sleep* 39, no. 9 (September 1, 2016): 1681–1690, https://doi.org/10.5665/sleep.6092

228 Kana Okano et al., "Sleep Quality, Duration, and Consistency Are Associated with Better Academic Performance in College Students," *Npj Science of Learning* 4, no. 1 (October 1, 2019): 1–5, https://doi.org/10.1038/s41539-019-0055-z

229 June C. Lo et al., "Neurobehavioral Impact of Successive Cycles of Sleep Restriction With and Without Naps in Adolescents," *Sleep* 40, no. 2 (February 1, 2017): zsw042, https://doi.org/10.1093/sleep/zsw042

230 Michigan Medicine—University of Michigan, "Irregular Sleep Schedules Connected to Bad Moods and Depression, Study Shows: The More Variation in Wake-up Time and Sleep Time, the Worse Mood and More Chance of Depression Symptoms in Study of First-Year Medical Residents," *ScienceDaily*, February 18, 2021, https://www.sciencedaily.com/releases/2021/02/210218094502.htm

231 Sean W. Cain et al., "Evening Home Lighting Adversely Impacts the Circadian System and Sleep," *Scientific Reports* 10, no. 1 (November 5, 2020): 19110, https://doi.org/10.1038/s41598-020-75622-4

232 "The Color of the Light Affects the Circadian Rhythms." Centers for Disease Control and Prevention. April 1, 2020. https://www.cdc.gov/niosh/emres/longhourstraining/color.html.

233 LaMotte, Sandee. "The Truth about White (and Pink and Brown) Noise for Sleep." CNN. Cable News Network, May 3, 2021. https://www.cnn.com/2021/03/18/health/white-pink-brown-noise-sleep-wellness/index.html.

234 Dave Philipps, "The Army Rolls Out a New Weapon: Strategic Napping," *The New York Times*, October 1, 2020, https://www.nytimes.com/2020/10/01/us/army-naps.html

235 Walker, *Why We Sleep*, 342.

236 Hillary Rowe et al., "The Curious Incident of the Dog in the Nighttime: The Effects of Pet-Human Co-Sleeping and Bedsharing on Sleep Dimensions of Children and Adolescents," *Sleep Health* 7, no. 3 (June 1, 2021): 324–331, https://doi.org/10.1016/j.sleh.2021.02.007

237 Rafael Pelayo, *How to Sleep: The New Science-Based Solutions for Sleeping Through the Night* (New York, NY: Artisan Books, a division of Workman Publishing Co., 2020), 136.

Chapter 12: What About Tech?

238 Monica Anderson and Jingjing Jiang, "Teens, Social Media & Technology 2018," *Pew Research Center*, May 31, 2018, https://www.pewresearch.org/internet/2018/05/31/teens-social-media-technology-2018/

239 Deirdre M. Harrington et al., "Concurrent Screen Use and Cross-Sectional Association with Lifestyle Behaviours and Psychosocial Health in Adolescent Females," *Acta Paediatrica* 110, no. 7 (February 11, 2021): 2164–2170, https://doi.org/10.1111/apa.15806

240 Monique K. LeBourgeois et al., "Digital Media and Sleep in Childhood and Adolescence," *Pediatrics* 140, no. S2 (November 1, 2017): S92–96, https://doi.org/10.1542/peds.2016-1758J

241 Ben Carter et al., "Association Between Portable Screen-Based Media Device Access or Use and Sleep Outcomes: A Systematic Review and Meta-Analysis," *JAMA Pediatrics* 170, no. 12 (December 1, 2016): 1202–1208, https://doi.org/10.1001/jamapediatrics.2016.2341

242 Jennifer D. Shapka, "Adolescent Technology Engagement: It Is More Complicated than a Lack of Self-Control," *Human Behavior and Emerging Technologies* 1, no. 2 (April 26, 2019): 103–110, https://doi.org/10.1002/hbe2.144

243 Björn Lindström et al., "A Computational Reward Learning Account of Social Media Engagement," *Nature Communications* 12, no. 1 (February 26, 2021): 1311, https://doi.org/10.1038/s41467-020-19607-x

244 Sharon Goulds et al., *Free to Be Online? Girls' and Young Women's Experiences of Online Harassment* (Plan International; Girls get Equal, 2020), https://plan-international.org/publications/freetobeonline

245 Shapka, "Adolescent Technology Engagement."

246 Daniel L. King et al., "The Impact of Prolonged Violent Video-Gaming on Adolescent Sleep: An Experimental Study," *Journal of Sleep Research* 22, no. 2 (2013): 137–143, https://doi.org/10.1111/j.1365-2869.2012.01060.x

247 Lauren Hale et al., "Youth Screen Media Habits and Sleep: Sleep-Friendly Screen Behavior Recommendations for Clinicians, Educators, and Parents," *Child and Adolescent Psychiatric Clinics of North America*, 27, no. 2 (April 1, 2018): 229–245, https://doi.org/10.1016/j.chc.2017.11.014

248 Zhenjiang Liao et al., "Prevalence of Internet Gaming Disorder and Its Association with Personality Traits and Gaming Characteristics Among Chinese Adolescent Gamers," *Frontiers in Psychiatry* 11 (2020): 598585, https://doi.org/10.3389/fpsyt.2020.598585

249 Liese Exelmans and den Bulck Jan Van, "Binge Viewing, Sleep, and the Role of Pre-Sleep Arousal," *Journal of Clinical Sleep Medicine* 13, no. 08 (August 15, 2017): 1001–1008, https://doi.org/10.5664/jcsm.6704

250 Kevin Westcott et al., "Digital Media Trends Survey: A New World of Choice for Digital Consumers," *Deloitte Insights*, March 20, 2018, https://www2.deloitte.com/us/en/insights/industry/technology/digital-media-trends-consumption-habits-survey-2018.html

251 Sidneyeve Matrix, "The Netflix Effect: Teens, Binge Watching, and On-Demand Digital Media Trends," *Jeunesse: Young People, Texts, Cultures* 6, no. 1 (May 21, 2014).

252 Bridget Rubenking et al., "Defining New Viewing Behaviours: What Makes and Motivates TV Binge-Watching?," *International Journal of Digital Television* 9, no. 1 (March 1, 2018): 69–85, https://doi.org/10.1386/jdtv.9.1.69_1

253 Exelmans and Van, "Binge Viewing, Sleep, and the Role of Pre-Sleep Arousal."

254 Sleep Junkies Podcast, "Screen Time and Sleep—It's Not All about Blue Light: Dr. Michael Grandner," March 31, 2020, in *Sleep Junkies,* podcast, EP43, https://sleepjunkies.com/screens-and-sleep/

255 Laurence D. Steinberg, *Age of Opportunity: Lessons from the New Science of Adolescence* (Boston: Houghton Mifflin Harcourt, 2015), 95.

256 Holly Scott, Stephany M. Biello, and Heather Cleland Woods, "Identifying Drivers for Bedtime Social Media Use Despite Sleep Costs: The Adolescent Perspective," *Sleep Health* 5, no. 6 (December 1, 2019): 539–545, https://doi.org/10.1016/j.sleh.2019.07.006

257 Sleep Junkies Podcast, "Screen Time and Sleep—It's Not All about Blue Light: Dr. Michael Grandner."

258 Jenny Bowler and Patrick Bourke, "Facebook Use and Sleep Quality: Light Interacts with Socially Induced Alertness," *British Journal of Psychology* 110, no. 3 (2019): 519–529, https://doi.org/10.1111/bjop.12351

259 Council on Communications and Media et al., "Media Use in School-Aged Children and Adolescents," *Pediatrics* 138, no. 5 (November 1, 2016): e20162592, https://doi.org/10.1542/peds.2016-2592

260 Carter et al., "Association Between Portable Screen-Based Media."

261 Nyissa A. Walsh et al., "Associations between Device Use before Bed, Mood Disturbance, and Insomnia Symptoms in Young Adults," *Sleep Health* 6, no. 6 (December 1, 2020): 822–827, https://doi.org/10.1016/j.sleh.2020.04.004

262 Dorit Shoval, Nama Tal, and Orna Tzischinsky, "Relationship of Smartphone Use at Night with Sleep Quality and Psychological Well-Being among Healthy Students: A Pilot Study," *Sleep Health* 6, no. 4 (August 1, 2020): 495–497, https://doi.org/10.1016/j.sleh.2020.01.011

263 Subramani Parasuraman et al., "Smartphone Usage and Increased Risk of Mobile Phone Addiction: A Concurrent Study," *International Journal of Pharmaceutical Investigation* 7, no. 3 (September 2017): 125–131, https://doi.org/10.4103/jphi.JPHI_56_17

264 National Sleep Foundation, "2014 Sleep in the Modern Family," *Sleep Foundation*, October 19, 2018, https://www.sleepfoundation.org/professionals/sleep-americar-polls/2014-sleep-modern-family

Chapter 13: How to Help Change School Start Times: Strategies for Success

265 Nicole G. Nahmod et al., "High School Start Times after 8:30 Am Are Associated with Later Wake Times and Longer Time in Bed Among Teens in a National Urban Cohort Study," *Sleep Health*, School Start Times, 3, no. 6 (December 1, 2017): 444–450, https://doi.org/10.1016/j.sleh.2017.09.004

266 June C. Lo et al., "Sustained Benefits of Delaying School Start Time on Adolescent Sleep and Well-Being," *Sleep* 41, no. 6 (June 2018), https://doi.org/10.1093/sleep/zsy052

267 "Homepage—Community Tool Box," *Community Tool Box*, https://ctb.ku.edu/en

268 "Resolution on Healthy Sleep for Adolescents," *National PTA*, https://www.pta.org/home/advocacy/ptas-positions/Individual-PTA-Resolutions/Resolution-on-Healthy-Sleep-for-Adolescents

269 Galit Levi Dunietz et al., "Later School Start Times: What Informs Parent Support or Opposition?," *Journal of Clinical Sleep Medicine* 13, no. 07 (July 15, 2017): 889–897, https://doi.org/10.5664/jcsm.6660

270 Lisa J Meltzer et al., "Changing School Start Times: Impact on Sleep in Primary and Secondary School Students," *Sleep* 44, no. 7 (July 1, 2021): zsab048, https://doi.org/10.1093/sleep/zsab048

271 Jan Hoffman, "To Keep Teenagers Alert, Schools Let Them Sleep In," *The New York Times*, March 13, 2014, sec. Well (Blog), https://well.blogs.nytimes.com/2014/03/13/to-keep-teenagers-alert-schools-let-them-sleep-in/

Chapter 14: How to Help Change School Start Times: Insights on What to Expect

272 Judith Owens et al., "School Start Time Change: An In-Depth Examination of School Districts in the United States," *Mind, Brain, and Education* 8, no. 4 (2014), https://doi.org/10.1111/mbe.12059

273 Susan Kohl Malone, Terra Ziporyn, and Alison M. Buttenheim, "Applying Behavioral Insights to Delay School Start Times," *Sleep Health*, School Start Times, 3, no. 6 (December 2017): 483–485, https://doi.org/10.1016/j.sleh.2017.07.012

274 Jeffrey A. Groen and Sabrina Wulff Pabilonia, "Snooze or Lose: High School Start Times and Academic Achievement," *Economics of Education Review* 72 (2019), https://doi.org/10.1016/j.econedurev.2019.05.011

275 Gideon P. Dunster et al., "Sleepmore in Seattle: Later School Start Times Are Associated with More Sleep and Better Performance in High School Students," *Science Advances* 4, no. 12 (December 1, 2018): eaau6200, https://doi.org/10.1126/sciadv.aau6200

276 Judith A. Owens et al., "A Quasi-Experimental Study of the Impact of School Start Time Changes on Adolescent Sleep," *Sleep Health* 3, no. 6 (December 2017): 437–443, https://doi.org/10.1016/j.sleh.2017.09.001

277 Rachel Widome et al., "Association of Delaying School Start Time with Sleep Duration, Timing, and Quality Among Adolescents," *JAMA Pediatrics* 174, no. 7 (July 1, 2020): 697–704, https://doi.org/10.1001/jamapediatrics.2020.0344

278 April Montgomery and Ken Mingis, "The Evolution of Apple's iPhone," *Computerworld*, September 23, 2021, https://www.computerworld.com/article/2604020/the-evolution-of-apples-iphone.html

279 Owens et al., "A Quasi-Experimental Study of the Impact of School Start Time."

280 Adolescent Sleep Working Group et al., "School Start Times for Adolescents," *Pediatrics* 134, no. 3 (September 2014), https://doi.org/10.1542/peds.2014-1697

281 Lisa L. Lewis, "Why Does High School Still Start So Early?," *Slate*, September 4, 2017, https://slate.com/technology/2017/09/stop-starting-school-before-8-30-a-m.html

Chapter 15: Later Start Times in California

282 Theresa Harrington, "State Legislature Approves Later Start Times for California Middle, High School Students," *EdSource*, September 14, 2019, https://edsource.org/2019/revised-bill-proposes-later-school-start-times-for-california-middle-high-school-students/616181

283 Mike McPhate, "California Today: Should the School Day Start Later?," *The New York Times*, August 2, 2017, https://www.nytimes.com/2017/08/02/us/california-today-school-start-time.html

Epilogue: Where We Are Today

284 Mary A. Carskadon, "Sleep in Adolescents: The Perfect Storm," *Pediatric Clinics of North America* 58, no. 3 (June 2011): 637–647, https://doi.org/10.1016/j.pcl.2011.03.003

ABOUT THE AUTHOR

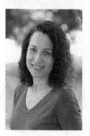

As a parenting journalist, Lisa L. Lewis has long covered a wide range of topics related to kids, public health, and education. After her 2016 *Los Angeles Times* op-ed spurred a California state bill on later secondary school start times, she quickly became immersed, playing a key role in the state's school start times law (the first of its kind in the nation).

Lewis has written for the *New York Times*, the *Atlantic*, the *Washington Post*, the *Los Angeles Times*, *Slate*, and *Your Teen*, among others. She's the parent of a teen and a recent teen, who inspire much of what she writes about—everything from concussions and heatstroke to school lockdowns to sleep. She lives in California.

www.lisallewis.com

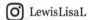 LewisLisaL

LewisLisaL

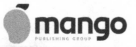

Mango Publishing, established in 2014, publishes an eclectic list of books by diverse authors—both new and established voices—on topics ranging from business, personal growth, women's empowerment, LGBTQ studies, health, and spirituality to history, popular culture, time management, decluttering, lifestyle, mental wellness, aging, and sustainable living. We were recently named 2019 *and* 2020's #1 fastest-growing independent publisher by *Publishers Weekly*. Our success is driven by our main goal, which is to publish high-quality books that will entertain readers as well as make a positive difference in their lives.

Our readers are our most important resource; we value your input, suggestions, and ideas. We'd love to hear from you—after all, we are publishing books for you!

Please stay in touch with us and follow us at:

Facebook: Mango Publishing
Twitter: @MangoPublishing
Instagram: @MangoPublishing
LinkedIn: Mango Publishing
Pinterest: Mango Publishing
Newsletter: mangopublishinggroup.com/newsletter

Join us on Mango's journey to reinvent publishing, one book at a time.

CPSIA information can be obtained
at www.ICGtesting.com
Printed in the USA
JSHW021541150622
27118JS00001B/55

9 781642 507911